Renal Diet Cookbook

Quick & Easy Low Phosphorus Recipes for People with Kidney Disease

By
Tara Sugar

Introduction

Your diet significantly influences your kidneys' health, so it is essential to consider which foods are better to consume and which ones can cause complications. The amount of protein, sodium, potassium, and phosphorus you eat is regulated by a proper renal diet. Following this diet can help lower the number of wastes your body absorbs, which can decrease your kidneys' workload and likely maintain the function of the kidneys. The renal diet can help keep the condition from advancing to the next level and prevent several years of complete renal failure or dialysis. Thinking about whether you can eat on a low-protein, low-sodium, low-potassium, and low-phosphorus diet can be very daunting. It's not as easy as making one small adjustment or cutting a few forms of foods from your diet. When you dine out, this book takes the surprise and tension out of finding out recipes, as well as what to select from the menu. Most notably, it will help you excel in the long-term management of lifestyle changes. A restrictive renal diet can be; you're not banished to years of bland foods.

In Chapter Five, the 28-day meal plan will help to get you started. Many of the recipes also make improvements to suit people or others undergoing dialysis with end-stage renal failure.

It is essential to equip yourself with information when it comes to a renal diet. In the days ahead, consider me to be your dietitian and cheerleader. Keep optimistic and do your best to commit to and above the 28-day program, and you will be on the road to better, happy kidneys. You're going to do it!

Chapter 1: How Kidneys Work And What Is Their Role In Our Systems?

Among the vital organs of the human body are the kidneys. Malfunctions of the kidneys may lead to severe illness or even death. Each kidney has a very complex function.

They have two essential purposes, in particular: to filter out poisonous and hazardous waste materials and to maintain the equilibrium of fluids, salts, water, and chemicals, i.e., electrolytes such as potassium, sodium, etc.

1.1. Anatomy of the Kidney

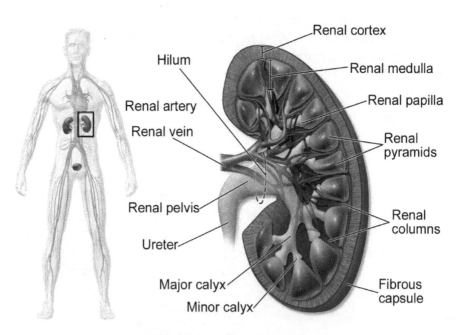

Kidney Anatomy

By removing excess water and hazardous waste materials from the bloodstream, the kidney produces urine.

Urine produced in each kidney passes through the ureter and flows through the urethra into the bladder until it is finally excreted.

Many individuals have two kidneys.

- On either side of the spine, the kidneys are positioned at the top and back of the

  abdomen. They are protected by the lower ribs from damage.

- Kidneys lie deep within the abdomen, so they cannot be felt naturally.

- A pair of bean-shaped organs are the kidneys. In an adult, a kidney is approximately 10 cm long, 4 cm thick, and 6 cm wide.

- Each kidney weights 150-170 grammes or so.

Urine processed in the kidneys filters down to the urinary bladder and then through the ureters. Each ureter is approximately 25 cm long and consists of special muscles in a hollow tube-like structure.

The urinary bladder is a hollow organ which consists of muscles that lie in the lower and anterior parts of the abdomen. It acts as a reservoir for urine.

The adult urinary bladder holds between 400-500 ml of urine; when filled to near full, a human experience the need to urinate. The urine in the bladder is excreted by the urethra throughout the urination process. In females, the urethra is comparatively small, whereas it is much longer in males.

Why are the kidneys essential for a living?

- Every day, we eat different forms and amounts and kinds of food.
- There are also regular differences in the number of salts, water, and acids in our bodies.

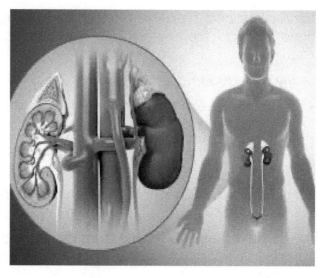

- The continuous process of transforming food into energy creates toxic chemicals that

  are unsafe.
- Such causes lead to changes in quantity of electrolytes, acids and electrolytes in the

  body. Accumulating unnecessary toxic substances can be life-threatening.
- The kidney works out the vital task of flushing out dangerous and poisonous by-products. They also preserve and control the proper equilibrium and quantities of acids, water, and electrolytes at the same time.

What are the functions of the kidney?

The kidney's primary function is to produce urine and purify the blood. Each kidney eliminates waste materials and other chemicals that the body does not need. Below are

the most important functions of the kidney.

1. Removal of waste products

- The most significant feature of the kidney is the purification of blood by eliminating waste materials.

- The food that we consume contains protein. For the growth and repair of the body, protein is needed. However, it produces waste materials as the body consumes protein. Accumulating and preserving these waste materials is similar to storing poison inside the body. Each kidney can philter the blood and radioactive waste products that are eventually excreted into the urine.

- The two important waste compounds that can easily be measured in the blood are urea and creatinine. "In blood testing, their "values reflect the function of the kidney. The blood test value of creatinine and urea would be high if both kidneys collapsed.

2. Removal of excess fluid

- The second most important kidney function is to regulate fluid equilibrium by excreting excess water as urine while storing the body's sufficient volume of water, crucial for life. They lose the potential to remove this surplus volume of water when the kidneys collapse. In the body, extra water results in swelling.

3. Balance Minerals and Chemicals

The kidneys play another important function of regulating minerals and chemicals like potassium, sodium, calcium, phosphorus, hydrogen, bicornate, and magnesium and maintain the normal composition of body fluid. Changes in the level of sodium can affect

the mental state of the person. In contrast, changes in potassium level can have significant adverse effects on heart rhythm and muscle functioning. Maintenance of a normal level of phosphorus and calcium is vital for healthy bones and teeth.

1.2. Control of Blood Pressure

The kidneys represent different hormones (renin, aldosterone, angiotensin, prostaglandin, etc.) that help control the body's salt and water, which play a key role in maintaining good blood pressure control. Hormone development and water regulation disruptions and salt in a patient with kidney disease can result in high blood pressure. Another hormone formed in the kidneys is erythropoietin, which plays a significant role in developing red blood cells. During kidney failure, erythropoietin production is diminished, leading to decreased RBC production, resulting in low hemoglobin production (anemia). It explains programs that run supplementation with iron and vitamin preparation. The hemoglobin count does not improve in patients with kidney disease And preserve strong bones. Vitamin D is processed into its active form by the kidneys, which is important for extracting calcium from food, developing teeth and bones, and preserving solid and stable bones. During kidney disease, diminished active vitamin D contributes to reduced and impaired development of the bones. In infants, growth retardation can be a symptom of kidney failure.

1.3. Chronic Kidney Disease (CKD)

Chronic kidney disease includes conditions that harm your kidneys and lessen their ability to keep you fit and active. If your kidney's condition gets worse, waste will build up to high levels in your blood and leave you feeling sick. It is possible to develop high blood

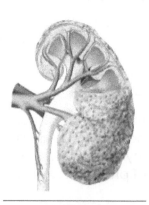

pressure, weak bones, inadequate diet nutrition, anemia (low blood count), and nerve damage. The risk of having heart and blood vessel disease is also increased by kidney disease. Over a long period, these problems can happen slowly.

Chronic kidney disease is usually caused by diabetes, high blood pressure, and other disorders. Chronic kidney disease will also be prevented from getting worse by treatment and early diagnosis. As kidney disease advances, it can ultimately lead to kidney failure, requiring dialysis or a kidney transplant to sustain life. Thirty-seven million Americans have Chronic Kidney Disease, and millions of others are at increased risk for Chronic Kidney Disease (CKD).

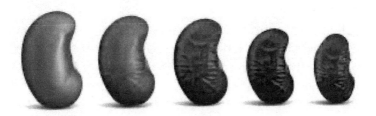

Chronic Kidney Disease (CKD)

Initial detection is crucial to prevent the progression of kidney disease towards kidney failure. Heart disease is the main cause of death for all individuals with CKD. The glomerular filtration rate is the best estimate of kidney function (GFR). CKD is triggered by high blood pressure, and CKD causes hypertension. Persistent proteinuria (urine protein) proves that there is CKD. Categories of high risk include those with hypertension, diabetes, and a history of kidney failure in the family. African Americans, Hispanics, Pacific Islanders, American Indians, and seniors are at higher risk. Two tests can detect CKD: blood pressure, serum creatinine, and albumin urine.

1.4. Understanding Kidney Disease

You will feel more empowered and less scared of having lived with the illness when you enlighten yourself regarding chronic kidney disease. You could take control of your life back! It is very important what you eat and the lifestyle choices you make. You can take many steps to prolong your kidney function if you are successfully treated in the disease's early stages. Chances are very good that you will be able to enjoy a high-quality, happy,

and active life when you make positive changes, have patience, and commit to working closely with your health care team.

1.5. Causes of CKD?

The two primary causes of chronic kidney disease are high blood pressure and diabetes. Up to two-thirds of the cases are due to them. When your blood sugar is too high, diabetes occurs, causing damage to many.

The body's organs, including the heart and kidneys, as well as blood vessels, eyes, and nerves. When your blood pressure against the walls of your blood vessels increases, hypertension, or high blood pressure, happens. If uncontrolled or poorly regulated, high blood pressure may be a leading cause of heart attacks, strokes, and chronic kidney disease. Also, high blood pressure can lead to chronic kidney disease. Other conditions that affect the kidneys are Glomerulonephritis, is a group of diseases that cause inflammation and deficiency of the kidney's filtering units. The third most frequent type of kidney disease is these disorders.

Hereditary diseases, such as polycystic kidney disease, cause large cysts to develop in the kidneys and destroy the surrounding tissue. Malformations happen when a baby grows in her mother's womb. A narrowing that prevents normal urine outflow and causes urine to flow back to the kidney, for example, may occur. It causes infections, and it is possible to damage the kidneys. Lupus and other illnesses affect the body's immune system. Blockages are caused by male disorders, such as kidney stones, tumors, or enlarged prostate glands. Frequent infections with urine.

1.6. Five Stages of Chronic Kidney Disease

STAGE	DESCRIPTION	GLOMERULAR FILTRATION RATE (GFR)
Normal kidney function	Healthy kidneys	90 mL/min or more
Stage 1	Kidney damage with normal or high GFR	90 mL/min or more
Stage 2	Kidney damage with mild decrease in GFR	60–89 mL/min
Stage 3	3 Moderate decrease in GFR	30–59 mL/min
Stage 4	Severe decrease in GFR	15–29 mL/min

Stage 5	Kidney failure	Less than 15 mL/min or receiving dialysis

1.7. What are the symptoms of CKD?

Most individuals do not have any significant symptoms until their kidney disease is advanced. However, you may realize that you:

- Have trouble concentrating
- Feel more tired and have less energy
- Have muscle cramping at night
- Have a poor appetite
- Have swollen feet and ankles
- Have trouble sleeping
- Have puffiness around your eyes, especially in the morning
- Need to urinate more often, especially at night.
- Have dry, itchy skin

At any age, any person can get chronic kidney disease. Some people are, however, more likely than others to develop kidney disease. If you have high blood pressure or diabetes are older with a family history of kidney failure belonging to a population group that has high blood pressure or a high rate of diabetes, such as Hispanic Americans, African Americans, Asian, American Indians, and Pacific Islanders, you could be at increased risk of developing kidney disease.

Chapter 2: Renal Diet Connection

Everyone needs to make good food decisions, but it is significantly essential to have chronic kidney disease. The making of safe food decisions has many advantages. A good diet gives you everyday life energy, stops illness, develops muscle, helps keep your weight stable, and can make your kidneys get weaker. Complications of kidney dysfunction, such as fluid pressure, high blood phosphorus, high blood potassium, bone disease, and weight loss, are avoided by proper diet.

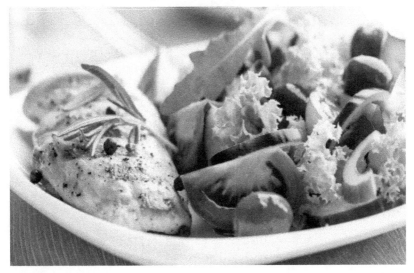

LOW PHOSPHORUS (Less than 150 mg/serving)	MEDIUM PHOSPHORUS (151–250 mg/serving)	HIGH PHOSPHORUS (More than 51 mg/serving)
Apple	Beans, black, 1 cup	Peanuts, oil roasted, 2 ounces
Bagel, 1 plain (4-inch diameter)	Beans, fava, 1 cup	Almonds, oil/dry roasted, 2 ounces
Barley, pearled, cooked	Beans, kidney, 1 cup	Baked beans, 1 cup
Beans, green	Beans, pinto, 1 cup	Beans, small white, mature, boiled, 1 cup
Bread, pita, 1 (6.5-inch diameter)	Beef, bottom round, 3 ounces	Beef, liver, cooked, 3 ounces
Bread, pumpernickel, 2 slices	Beef, chuck roast, 3 ounces	Beefalo, 3 ounces
Butter, 1 tablespoon	Beef, eye round, 3 ounces	Buttermilk, 1 cup
Cabbage	Beef, ground, 70% lean, 3 ounces	Calamari, fried, 3 ounces
Cauliflower	Beef, ground, 95% lean, 3 ounces	Cashews, dry roasted, 2 ounces
Cereal, crispy rice, 1 cup	Beef, sirloin steak, 3	Cereal, bran, 100%

	ounces		2.1.
Cheese, Brie, 1 ounce	Black-eyed peas, 1 cup	Cereal, wheat germ, ¼ cup	**Key**
Cheese, feta, 1 ounce	Bread, whole wheat, 2 slices	Cheese, goat, 2 ounces	
Cocoa, unsweetened, 2 tablespoons	Catfish, breaded/fried, 3 ounces	Cheese, parmesan, 2 ounces	

Diet Concerns

Your "prescription" renal diet can range depending on the level of your kidney failure, the form of medication, the outcome of blood tests, and whether you have diabetes or elevated blood pressure. It can at first sound overwhelming to adopt a renal diet, but it is easier to follow than expected. This book, the 28-day diet plan outlined, will give you a fantastic start and deliver you tasty, kidney-friendly recipes in this book.

The below very essential macronutrients, vitamins, and minerals are outlined in this section, which should be carefully monitored to keep your kidneys as healthy as possible:

- **Potassium**
- **Phosphorus Calories**
- **Protein Fats Sodium**
- **Carbohydrates**
- **Vitamins/Minerals**
- **Fluids**

Bear in mind when you read this book that serving size is the bottom line on whether a meal is medium, moderate, or heavy in a given nutrient. For instance, a low-potassium diet has become a high-potassium serving of that food if you consume a big bowl of raspberries instead of a half-cup serving.

Potassium

To keep the heart healthy and Strong, Potassium is an essential mineral that the body requires. Holding the water balance between your cells and body fluids in place is also important. By urination, good kidneys expel excess potassium. If the kidneys do not function well, potassium cannot be absorbed, building up in the blood.

It may be dangerous for the body to get too much or too little potassium in the blood. Although more potassium is required for certain individuals with kidney failure, others require less. Depending on how well your kidneys perform, your need for potassium can differ.

There is some potassium in all diets, but some foods contain significant quantities of potassium. A table that lists low-potassium, medium potassium, and high-potassium foods is on the following pages. The amount of potassium you ingest is typically not reduced if you have chronic kidney disease unless your blood potassium content is high. Please speak to your doctor about testing your potassium level in your blood. And your potassium intake should be maintained between 2,000 and 3,000 milligrams a day while you are undergoing dialysis.

2.2. Phosphorus in Common Foods

Calories

Among all things that we ingest, calories are existed and give us the energy to work daily. When you have kidney disease, your calorie needs are higher, especially if you're on dialysis. You could be suggested to modify your diet if you have phase 3 or 4 chronic kidney disease, especially if you are not at a healthy weight. Depending on the health, you might be advised to gain or lose a few pounds. Maintaining a positive appetite will help you treat your kidney disease and avoid more complications with your kidneys. With a balanced weight-loss regime, blood pressure and blood sugar levels normally increase. It can postpone or avoid further kidney damage.

If you need to add calories to your diet to raise the weight, adding one high-fat item to meals or snacks is the easiest way to do this. In the "Fats" portion of this chapter, several healthy-fat food choices are listed (here). Regular calorie requirements are 30 to 35 calories per kilogram of body weight, in both chronic kidney failure and with dialysis. So, if you weigh 150 pounds a day, that's about 2,000 calories.

Protein

In the body, protein plays a very important function. To repair tissues, build muscles, and battle infection, your body requires protein. That is why it's so important to eat protein to remain healthy. Per day the average human requires between 40 and 65 grams of protein. Your protein consumption will be reduced to 12 to 15 percent of your calorie intake per day if you are in phases 1, 2, or 3 of chronic kidney disease, the same amount

recommended for a balanced diet for normal adults by the Dietary Guide Intakes (DRIs). Your protein consumption will be limited to 10 percent of your caloric intake if you are in stage 4 of chronic kidney disease.

It also extracts protein as dialysis cleans out waste from the blood. That's why you must consume enough protein to substitute for what's missing. Otherwise, the protein from your

muscles will start to be used by your body to get the protein it wants. It will cause you to lose weight, feel very weak, and raise the chance of being sick.

Around 1.2 grams of protein per kilogram of body weight per day can be consumed by people undergoing dialysis. In other words, it's around 82 grams of protein a day if you weigh 150 pounds. At least half of the protein you consume can come from protein products of good quality. It will make your kidneys function longer by keeping track of how much protein you consume. In curing the infection and repairing wounds, protein also plays a part, and it provides the body with a supply of energy. Here is a list of high-protein ingredients that can be used in your diet.

2.3. Common High-Protein Foods*

MEATS, POULTRY, DAIRY, AND EGGS:

- Beef, ground, 5% fat
- Beef, rib, lean, roasted
- Beef, bottom round
- Chicken, breast, without skin
- Chicken, dark meat, without skin
- Cod, Pacific
- Duck, cooked, without skin
- Flounder
- Halibut, Atlantic/Pacific
- Pollock
- Pork, leg, lean, roasted
- Pork chops
- Salmon, Atlantic
- Swordfish
- Tuna, light, canned in oil
- Tuna, yellowfin

- Tuna salad, 16.5 grams
- Veal, rib, lean, roasted
- Cheese, cottage, creamed
- Cheese, cottage, 2% fat
- Cheese, ricotta, part skim milk
- Cheese, ricotta, whole milk
- Egg substitute, ¼ cup, 6.0 grams
- Egg whole, 1 large, 6.2 grams
- Milk, dry, nonfat
- Yogurt, Greek, plain, nonfat, ⅔
- cup, 11 grams Yogurt, plain, low
- fat, 13 grams

LEGUMES, NUTS, GRAINS, AND CEREALS:

- Almonds, 2 ounces
- Cashews, dry roasted, 2 ounces
- Hazelnuts
- Peas, split, boiled, 1 cup
- Pine nuts, dried
- Pistachios, dry roasted
- Walnuts, English, chopped
- Lentils, boiled, 1 cup
- Beans, white, boiled, 1 cup
- Peanuts, dry roasted
- Soybeans, mature, boiled
- Bagel (4-inch diameter)
- Bread crumbs, 1 cup
- Wheat flour, white, 1 cup
- Wheat flour, whole grain, 1 cup

* One serving of meat = 3 ounces, delivering, unless otherwise mentioned, at least 20 grams of protein.

One serving of dairy = 1 cup, providing, unless otherwise stated, at least 20 grams of protein.

All the rest, one serving = 1/2 cup, containing, unless otherwise mentioned, at least 10 grams of protein.

Fats

If your blood lipid (fat) levels are high, you may need to cut down on the amount of fat you eat. There is an association between chronic kidney disease and heart disease. An increased risk of heart disease is related to your kidney disease and, typically, to other diabetes and high blood pressure problems. It is best to eat healthy fats like olive or canola oil. If your blood potassium and phosphorus levels are low enough to allow it, I recommend adding avocados, nuts, and seeds to your diet. Tuna and salmon also contain heart-healthy fats that make a good addition to your diet. The key is to keep your

fat intake to less than 30 percent of your daily calories. For example, if your calorie allowance is 2,000 calories, your calories from fat should be limited to 600 calories or about 70 grams of fat.

Sodium

Sodium is a mineral that helps control the water content and blood pressure of your body. Good kidneys can extract sodium from the body if required, but sodium can build up and cause high blood pressure, fluid weight gain, and thirst when the kidneys do not function properly. The risk of your kidney condition getting worse is raised by high blood pressure. If you are in the early stages of progressive kidney disease (stages 1 to 4), if you have elevated blood pressure or hold urine, you will need to make certain nutritional changes. You would need to adopt a low-sodium diet and not eat more than 1,500 milligrams of sodium per day equal to a little less than 1-teaspoon of salt if you have stage 5 chronic kidney disease need dialysis. (It is important to remember that 1-teaspoon of salt a day is the highest amount of sodium allowed, which covers all foods plus additional salt.) To keep the blood pressure under control, adopt a sodium-restricted diet carefully. Blood pressure management will also prevent the chances of contracting heart failure and reduce the probability that your kidney disease will worsen.

2.4. High-Sodium Foods to Avoid

- Table salt
- Seasoning salt
- Soy sauce
- Teriyaki sauce
- Garlic salt
- Onion salt
- Spam
- Vegetable juices
- Barbecue sauce
- Monosodium glutamate (MSG)
- Most canned foods
- Ham
- Salt pork
- Microwave meals
- Potato chips

- Salted crackers
- Buttermilk
- Canned ravioli
- Bouillon cubes
- Canned soups
- Sauerkraut
- Fast foods
- Salad dressings
- Hot dogs
- Cold cuts, deli meat
- Corned beef
- Frozen prepared foods
- Bacon

Chapter 3: Managing Your Renal Diet When You Are Diabetic

Diets are one of the most important therapies in the treatment of kidney disease and diabetes. If you have been diagnosed with kidney disease due to diabetes, you will need to consult with a dietician to build an eating routine that's good for you. This technique would help control blood glucose levels and reduce the amount of waste and fluid that the kidneys process.

3.1. Which nutrients do I need to regulate?

Your nutritionist will supply you with nutritional guidelines to tell you how much you will eat protein, fat, and carbohydrates and how much you can consume each day with phosphorus, sodium, and potassium. As these minerals need to be lower in your diet, you can limit or exclude certain foods when preparing your meals.

Control of sections is also important. Talk with your nutritionist about tips for correctly calculating a serving amount. What can be measured as one serving on a normal diet can be counted as three portions of the kidney.

The doctor and dietitian would also prescribe that you take meals and beverages of the same size and carbohydrate/calorie quality during some hours of the day to control the

blood glucose at an even amount. Blood glucose levels must still be monitored, and the doctor shares the findings.

3.2. What can I eat?

Below is an example of food options that are often prescribed on a regular renal diabetic diet. The use of foods containing sodium, phosphorus, potassium, and high sugar content is the subject of this list. Ask your nutritionist if you should get any of the foods described to make sure you understand what the recommended serving size should be. Carbohydrate Milk and Non-Milk Diets.

RECOMMENDED:

- Non-dairy creamer, plain yogurt, skim or fat-free milk, sugar-free pudding, sugar-free ice cream, sugar-free yogurt, sugar-free nondairy frozen desserts*

- Portions of dairy products are often limited to four ounces due to high potassium, phosphorus or protein content

AVOID:

- Buttermilk, sweetened yogurt, chocolate milk, sugar sweetened, sugar sweetened ice cream, pudding, sugar sweetened nondairy frozen desserts

3.3. Breads and starches

RECOMMENDED:

- Sourdough, whole grain bread and whole wheat, unsweetened, white, wheat, rye, cream of wheat, grits, malt-o-meal, rice, bagel (small), refined dry cereals, noodles, white or whole wheat pasta, cornbread (made from scratch), flour tortilla, hamburger bun, unsalted cracker.

AVOID:

Frosted or sugar-coated cereals, bran bread, gingerbread, pancake mix, cornbread mix, instant cereals, bran or granola, biscuits, salted snacks including: potato chips, corn chips and crackers Whole wheat cereals like oatmeal, wheat flakes and raisin bran, and whole

grain hot cereals contain more potassium and phosphorus than refined products.

3.4. Fruits and Juices

RECOMMENDED:

- Applesauce, apricot halves, apples, apple juice, berries including: cranberries, blackberries and blueberries, strawberries, raspberries, low sugar cranberry juice, grapes, grape juice, kumquats, cherries, fruit cocktail, grapefruit, plums, tangerine, watermelon, mandarin oranges, pears, pineapple, fruit canned in unsweetened juice

AVOID:

- Bananas, cantaloupe, avocados, dried fruits including: raisins, dates, and prunes, kumquats, star fruit, fresh pears, honeydew melon, kiwis, mangos, oranges and orange juice, papaya, nectarines, pomegranate, fruit canned in syrup

3.5. Starchy vegetables

RECOMMENDED:

- Mixed vegetables with corn and peas (eat these less often because they are high in phosphorus), corn, peas, potatoes (soaked to reduce potassium)

AVOID:

- Yams, baked beans, baked potatoes, sweet potatoes, dried beans (kidneys, pinto or soy, lima, lentil), succotash, winter squash, pumpkin

3.6. Non-starchy vegetables

RECOMMENDED:

- Brussels sprouts, carrots, asparagus, beets, broccoli, cabbage, cauliflower, celery, cucumber, green beans, iceberg lettuce, eggplant, frozen broccoli cuts, kale, leeks, red

AVOID:

- Beet greens, cactus, cooked Chinese cabbage, Artichoke, fresh bamboo shoots,
- kohlrabi, rutabagas, tomatoes, tomato and green peppers, mustard greens, okra, onions, radishes, raw spinach (1/2 cup), summer squash, turnips, snow peas, sauce or paste, sauerkraut, cooked spinach, tomato juice, vegetable juice

3.7. Higher-protein foods Meats, cheeses and eggs

RECOMMENDED:

- Lean cuts of meat, fish, poultry, and seafood; eggs, low cholesterol egg substitute; cottage cheese (limited due to high sodium content)

AVOID:

- Bacon, cheeses, hot dogs, canned and luncheon meats, organ meats, salami, salmon, sausage, nuts, pepperoni

3.8. Higher-fat foods Seasoning and calories

RECOMMENDED:

- Tub or soft margarine low in trans fats, cream cheese, low fat mayonnaise, mayonnaise, sour cream, low fat cream cheese, low fat sour cream

AVOID:

Bacon fat, Crisco®, lard, shortening, back fat, butter, margarines high in trans fats, whipping cream

3.9. Beverages

RECOMMENDED:

Water, diet clear sodas, lemonade sweetened or homemade tea with an artificial sweetener

AVOID:

Regular or diet dark colas, fruit-flavored drinks or water sweetened with fruit juices, syrup, or phosphoric acid; tea or lemonade sweetened with real sugar beer, fruit juices, bottled or lemonade containing sugar or canned iced tea.

You may also be instructed to avoid or limit the following salty and sweet foods:

- Honey
- Molasses
- Baked goods
- Candy
- Canned foods
- Condiments
- Onion, garlic or table salt
- Chocolate
- Regular sugar

- Syrup Ice cream
- TV dinners
- Meat tenderizer
- Salted chips and snacks
- Marinades
- Nuts Pizza

Chapter 4: Basics of Renal Diet

Eating enough is important for kidney function. Specifically, patients with kidney disease need to monitor their consumption of sodium, potassium, and phosphorus. Many important micronutrients may need to be treated by individuals with kidney disease as well.

The following details will motivate you to improve your diet. Speak about your specific and special diet criteria with your dietitian or doctor. Some of the compounds that are important for regulating or supporting a renal diet are:

4.1. Sodium

A mineral (sodium chloride) present in salt is called Sodium. Food production would be nothing without its inclusion since it is one of the seasonings most often used, and it takes time to adjust and reduce the salt in the food. Reducing salt/sodium, however, is an important aid in the treatment of kidney disease.

The presence of Sodium in the body. In most ways, people seem to believe that Sodium and salt are synonymous. Salt, however, is a complex of Sodium and chloride. There may be iodine in the food we eat, or there may be other forms of Sodium. Refined foods

contain larger sodium levels due to added iodine. Sodium is one of the body's three main

electrolytes (the other two being potassium and chloride). Electrolytes track the fluids flowing into and out of the tissues and cells of the body. Regulating blood supply and blood pressure Regulating muscle contraction and nerve function, Balancing the blood acid-base balance by regulating how much fluid the body loses or maintains.

How Sodium intake can be monitored?

Make sure you read the product labels. The sodium content is still mentioned. Preventing foods that contain more than 300 mg of Sodium per serving (or 600 mg for a full frozen meal). Avoid salt-containing foods with the first four or five products on the commodity list. In comparison to frozen meats, they select fresh ones. Be mindful of serving sizes well. Avoid consuming processed ingredients. Pick frozen or fresh fruit and veggies with a no salt added" sticker, and canned. Pick spices that do not list "salt" in their description (choose garlic powder instead of garlic salt). To use the smallest sodium parts, compare goods. Limit the average amount of Sodium per meal to 400 mg and 150 mg per snack. Don't use salt when cooking rice. Don't bring salt on rice while you're eating. It is not healthy to eat ham, pork, hot dogs, sausage, tea, chicken, or regular condensed soup. Produce only soups with labels indicating a drop in salt level and eat only one cup, not the entire can. "No salt added" is meant to mean canned vegetables.

Do not use seasoned salts, such as onion salt, garlic salt, or 'seasoned' salt. Even avoid the sea or koshe salt. Be sure you look for lower salt or no added salt substitutes for your preferred ingredients, such as box mixes or peanut butter. Do not buy frozen or refrigerated meats that are in a solution," canned or pre-seasoned." Usually, these things are pork chops, pork tenderloin, chicken breasts, burgers, or steaks."

4.2. Potassium

Potassium is a mineral involved in the functioning of muscles. When the kidneys don't work right, potassium builds up in the blood. It will induce changes in how the heartbeats, perhaps even progressing to a cardiac arrest. In vegetables and fruits, potassium is mainly present, plus meat and milk. Some of them would like to stop and limit the number of

others.

Potassium-rich foods to avoid:

Grapefruit juice, Prune juice, Bananas Citrus, and orange juice Peppers, tomato sauce, tomato juice, Pumpkin Winter squash Dried beans-all sorts of cooked vegetables, collards, Swiss Chard, spinach, kale Other things to avoid granola, molasses, bran cereals, "salt replacement" or "lite" salt.

Potatoes and sweet potatoes require special handling to allow you to eat them in SMALL doses. Peel them, break them into thin slices or cubes, and soak them over several hours in a large volume of water. When you are about to cook them and use a decent amount of water in the pan, drain the soaking water. Drain the water before you prepare them for feeding. Be sure to eat a wide variety of fruits and vegetables every day to prevent consuming too much potassium.

What is potassium in the body and its role?

In many of the foods we eat, potassium is a mineral present naturally found in the body. Potassium plays a crucial part in keeping the heartbeat normal and the organs working properly. Potassium is also necessary for the maintenance of water and electrolyte equilibrium in the bloodstream. The kidneys tend to retain potassium in the body adequately and eliminate excess quantities from the urine. How do kidney patients regulate their potassium intake? When the kidneys malfunction, they can no longer extract excess potassium, so potassium levels build up in the body. Hyperkalemia is known as fast potassium in the blood, which can cause:

- An irregular heartbeat
- Slow pulse
- Heart attacks
- Muscle weakness
- Death

How can patients monitor their potassium consumption?

A patient must monitor the amount of potassium that reaches the body when the kidneys no longer regulate potassium. Tips to help keep potassium levels in your blood safe: Speak to a renal dietitian about developing an eating routine. Reduce the consumption of food that is high in potassium. Limit the quantity to 8oz for dairy and milk products. Every day. Avoid potassium seasonings and sodium equivalents. Read stickers on packaged products to prevent potassium chloride. Keep on to your food log. For serving, pay attention to the size.

4.3. Phosphorus

Phosphorus is another mineral that will build up in your blood when your kidneys do not function properly. Calcium can be drained from your bones as this occurs and can settle into your skin or blood vessels. Bone illness will then become a challenge, making you more likely to get a crack in the bone.

Dairy foods are the main phosphorus source in the diet, so limit milk to one cup daily if you use cheese or yogurt instead of powdered milk, either one bottle OR one ounce a day! In certain fruits, there is also phosphorus. Limit them per WEEK to one cup of greens, broccoli, dried beans, sprouts, and fungi. Those cereals must be limited to one serving a week: wheat cereals, bran, granola, and oatmeal. White bread is better than bread or crackers made from whole grains. Phosphorus is also found in soft drinks, so only drink clear ones. Do not eat beverages.

Potassium and its role in the body?

Phosphorus is a mineral significant in the stabilization and growth of bones. Phosphorus also helps to grow connective tissue and organs and aids in the operation of muscles. The tiny intestines remove phosphorus to be stored in the bones as food containing phosphorus is ingested and digested.

Why do kidney patients monitor phosphorus intake?

Extra phosphorus can be drained from the blood by the kidneys that usually function. The

kidneys no longer expel excess phosphorus as kidney function is compromised. Large

---

amounts of phosphorus will drain the bones out of calcium, making them brittle. It also exists in the poisonous blood vessels, skin, lungs, and heart at calcium concentrations.

How are patients supposed to monitor their phosphorus intake?

Phosphorus can be present in some foods. Therefore, patients with impaired kidney function should work with a renal dietician to help regulate phosphorus levels. Tools to help retain phosphorus at safe levels:

1. Learn what low-phosphorus diets are.
2. Eat small amounts of food for meals and snacks that are rich in protein.
3. Pay careful attention to the scale of portions.
4. Eat fruits and vegetables that are fresh.
5. Warn the doctor of using phosphate binders at mealtime.
6. Avoid packaged foods that contain extra phosphorus.
7. Check for the words with "Look for the words on ingredient labels with " Keep on to your food log.

Nutrition, with healthy kidneys, is not a problem. Normally, protein is absorbed, and waste products are produced, which are filtered by the kidney's nephrons. Then the waste turns into the urine with the aid of additional renal proteins. On the other hand, weakened kidneys refuse to eliminate protein waste, and it builds up in the blood. For Chronic Kidney Disease patients, adequate protein intake is tricky as the amount varies with each disease stage. Protein is essential for maintaining tissues and other bodily functions, so it is critical to consume the prescribed amount for the particular degree of illness, according to the renal dietician or nephrologist.

Fluids:

There is also reduced urinary output in people on dialysis, so increased fluid in the body can place undue pressure on the person's heart and lungs. Based on the production of urine and dialysis conditions, the fluid allocation of a patient is calculated individually.

Following your nephrologist/fluid nutritionist's intake guidelines is critical.

Patients should follow these steps: Do not drink more than recommended by the doctor to regulate fluids intake. Count all foods that will melt, beware of the number of fluids involved in cooking at room temperature.

4.4. What is a Renal Diet?

Renal is a medical word that refers to the kidneys. Therefore, a renal diet is also known as a diet for dialysis or a kidney diet. It is a form of diet that improves the kidney's function and can help to slow the onset of complete kidney failure or even help prevent kidney failure from occurring. In a nutshell, blood includes waste materials from cells, drinks, and food that we consume and eat. And then, these wastes are washed out of the blood and expelled into the urine. The aim is to minimize the amount of waste in the blood when you have kidney disease and hence the value of adhering to a renal diet.

4.5. Essential Things You Need to Know About the Renal Diet

Now that you have an idea of how the kidneys work, it is easier to understand how it can be affected by food and diet. So here are some important details about this diet.

Sodium

Sodium is a mineral salt that is naturally present in foods. A particular sodium level is found in each food, and certain foods have higher levels of sodium than others. In general, salt or table salt is a chemical mixture of two minerals known as sodium chloride, their chemical name. The sodium and chloride ions can be broken into two separate ions. On the other side, packaged foods, regardless of the salt used for seasoning or preservative, have a higher-than-average sodium level.

Sodium in the body is among the top three main electrolytes used. Chloride and potassium are the two other electrolytes. In transferring fluids in and out of each cell of the body, electrolytes support. In specific, sodium helps control the volume of fluid to be stored or flushed out to regulate the blood's acid-base balance and regulate muscle movement and nerve activity. And lastly, it also helps control the volume and blood pressure of the blood.

Too much salt in the diet is not beneficial for the kidneys since it no longer functions efficiently to remove extra fluid and excess sodium from the body until it has a crisis. Thus, the need to log sodium intake.

The consumption of sodium in the renal diet does not exceed 150-mg per snack and 400-

mg per meal. So that's a limit of 1,350-mg one-snack sodium a day or 1,600-mg two-snack sodium.

The key to lessening sodium intake is by:

- Choosing fresh fruits and veggies
- No processed foods and eating out
- It is always best to cook your food using spices without added salt
- Not adding salt to your cooked food.
- Always use fresh food.

4.6. What to Do in a Renal Diet?

Eat more new fruits and vegetables such as apples, cranberries, oranges, pineapples and strawberries, cauliflower, onions, peppers, radishes, summer squash, and lettuce Pita, tortillas and white bread Italian white rice, fish and chicken, French or sourdough bread Corn or rice cereals and wheat cream.

4.7. Benefits of a Renal Diet

Patients can help prolong their kidneys' survival or life by undergoing a renal diet by not adding undue stress. You reduce their activity by encouraging the kidneys not to clean out and wash out ammonia, protein metabolites, wastewater, sodium, and potassium. Perhaps most significantly, as most healthcare experts would claim, avoidance is safer than therapy. It will also encourage a normal person like you and me to go on a kidney diet or renal diet to ensure the kidney failure is not right in our corner.

Chapter 5: 28-Day Renal Diet Meal Plan

In this Chapter we will discuss a 28-day meal plan, which is meant to take some of the guesswork out of preparing your menus and ingredient shopping. The grocery lists contain everything you need for the week to make breakfast, lunch, and dinner, but remember that no snack items are mentioned. You should have those ingredients until you know which snacks you want to have on hand. There may already be some items on the grocery lists in your pantry, so take a look at the amounts required for the week and buy an ingredient if you need it. If you make a pot of chicken broth in the first week, you can freeze it for the remainder of the meal plan in 1-cup amounts to use. If you have leftovers from every meal, replace them later in the week as a snack or another meal in the meal schedule.

The consumption of protein for each day varies between 35 and 50 grams, so add high-protein snacks or raise the portion sizes of high-protein dishes if you need more protein in your diet. Consult a licensed dietitian when in doubt to ensure that the individual needs are fulfilled.

Week 1 Meal Plan

Monday:

Breakfast: Mixed-Grain Hot Cereal

Lunch: Traditional Chicken-Vegetable Soup

Dinner: Baked Cod with Cucumber-Dill Salsa

Tuesday:

Breakfast: Corn Pudding

Lunch: Crab Cakes with Lime Salsa

Dinner: Pesto Pork Chops

Wednesday:

Breakfast: Fruit and Cheese Breakfast Wrap

Lunch: Linguine with Roasted Red Pepper–Basil Sauce

Dinner: Herb Pesto Tuna

Thursday:

Breakfast: Cinnamon-Nutmeg Blueberry Muffins

Lunch: Egg White Frittata with Penne

Dinner: Lemon-Herb Chicken

Friday:

Breakfast: Egg-in-the-Hole

Lunch: Five-Spice Chicken Lettuce Wraps

Dinner: Sweet Glazed Salmon

Saturday:

Breakfast: Skillet-Baked Pancake

Lunch: Turkey-Bulgur Soup

Dinner: Grilled Steak with Cucumber-Cilantro Salsa

Sunday:

Breakfast: Strawberry–Cream Cheese Stuffed French Toast

Lunch: Couscous Burgers

Dinner: Indian Chicken Curry

Suggested Snacks:

Cinnamon Applesauce, Blueberry-Pineapple Smoothie, Spicy Kale

Chips, Hard-boiled eggs

Grapes

Ice pops

Rice cakes

Week 1 Shopping List

Fruits and Vegetables

- Apples (2)
- Blueberries (8 ounces)
- Cabbage, green, shredded (½ cup)
- Carrots (4)
- Celery stalks (7)
- Corn, frozen kernels (2 cups)
- Cucumbers, English (2)
- Garlic (16 cloves, or 9 teaspoons minced and 4 cloves)
- Jalapeño pepper (1)
- Lemons (4)
- Lettuce, Boston (1 head)
- Limes (4)
- Onions, sweet (5)
- Peppers, bell, red (2)
- Scallions (4)
- Snow peas (½ cup)
- Sprouts, bean (½ cup)

Dairy and Dairy Alternatives

- Butter, unsalted (¾ cup)
- Cheese, cream, plain (5 ounces)
- Cheese, Parmesan, low-fat (1 ounce)
- Eggs (18 eggs)
- Milk, coconut (¼ cup)
- Milk, unsweetened rice (4½ cups)
- Milk, vanilla, rice, not enriched (1¼ cups)

- Sour cream, light (2 tablespoons)

Spices and Herbs

- Basil, fresh (2 bunches)
- Bay leaves, dried (4)
- Cardamon, ground
- Cayenne pepper
- Chinese five-spice powder
- Chives, fresh (1 bunch)
- Cilantro, fresh (1 bunch)
- Cinnamon, ground
- Cloves, ground
- Coriander, ground
- Cumin, ground
- Curry powder
- Dill, fresh (1 bunch)
- Fennel powder
- Ginger, fresh (2-inch piece) Ginger, ground
- Green chili powder
- Mustard, ground
- Nutmeg, ground
- Oregano, fresh (1 bunch)
- Parsley, fresh (1 bunch)
- Peppercorns, black, freshly ground Peppercorns, black
- Red pepper flakes
- Sage, fresh (1 bunch)
- Sweet paprika, ground
- Thyme, fresh (1 bunch)
- Turmeric, ground

Fish and Seafood

- Cod (4 fillets totaling 12 ounces)
- Crab meat, queen (8 ounces)
- Salmon (4 fillets totaling 12 ounces)
- Shrimp (8 ounces)
- Tuna, yellowfin (4 fillets totaling 12 ounces)

Meat and Poultry

- Beef, tenderloin (4 steaks totaling 12 ounces)
- Chicken breasts, boneless, skinless
- (36 ounces)
- Chicken carcass, skin removed (1)
- Chicken thighs, boneless, skinless (6) Pork, top loin (4 chops totaling 12 ounces)
- Turkey, ground, 93% lean (8 ounces)

Other

- Baking soda substitute, Ener-G (3½ teaspoons) Bread, Italian (2 slices) Bread, white (8 slices)
- Bread crumbs
- Buckwheat, whole (2 tablespoons) Bulgur (½ cup)
- Chickpeas (4 ounces)
- Cooking spray
- Couscous (2 cups)
- Flour, all-purpose
- Honey
- Hot pepper sauce
- Jam, strawberry (¼ cup)
- Linguine
- Oil, canola

- Oil, olive
- Penne
- Sugar, granulated
- Tortillas, flour, 6-inch diameter (2) Vanilla extract, pure
- Vinegar, apple cider
- Vinegar, balsamic

Week 2 Meal Plan

Monday:

Breakfast: Fruit and Cheese Breakfast Wrap

Lunch: Indian Chicken Curry

Dinner: Classic Pot Roast

Tuesday:

Breakfast: Mixed-Grain Hot Cereal

Lunch: Roasted Beef Stew

Dinner: Sweet Glazed Salmon

Wednesday:

Breakfast: Cinnamon-Nutmeg Blueberry Muffins

Lunch: Couscous Burgers

Dinner: Persian Chicken

Thursday:

Breakfast: Egg-in-the-Hole

Lunch: Five-Spice Chicken Lettuce Wraps

Dinner: Baked Cod with Cucumber-Dill Salsa

Friday:

Breakfast: Corn Pudding

Lunch: Traditional Chicken-Vegetable Soup

Dinner: Sweet and Sour Meat Loaf

Saturday:

Breakfast: Strawberry–Cream Cheese Stuffed French Toast

Lunch: Egg White Frittata with Penne

Dinner: Pesto Pork Chops

Sunday:

Breakfast: Skillet-Baked Pancake

Lunch: Linguine with Roasted Red Pepper–Basil Sauce

Dinner: Herb Pesto Tuna

Suggested Snacks:

Cooked Four-Pepper Salsa with baked pita wedges, Apple-Chai Smoothie, Meringue Cookies, Tuna salad

Apple

Unsalted popcorn

Watermelon

Week 2 Shopping List

Fruits and Vegetables

- Apples (2)
- Blueberries (8 ounces)
- Carrots (4)
- Celery stalks (8)
- Corn, frozen kernels (2 cups)
- Cucumber, English (1)
- Garlic (14 cloves or 10 teaspoons minced and 2 cloves)
- Lemons (4)
- Lettuce, Boston (1 head)

- Limes (2)
- Onions, sweet (6)
- Peppers, banana (2)
- Peppers, bell, red (2)
- Pepper, bell, green (1)
- Pepper, jalapeño (2)
- Scallion (2)
- Snow peas (½ cup)
- Sprouts, bean (½ cup)

Dairy and Dairy Alternatives

- Butter, unsalted (½ cup)
- Cheese, Parmesan, low-fat (1 ounce)
- Cheese, cream, plain (5 ounces)
- Eggs (18)
- Sour cream, light (2 tablespoons)
- Milk, coconut (¼ cup)
- Milk, rice, unsweetened (4 cups)
- Milk, rice, vanilla (1¼ cups)

Spices and Herbs

- Basil, fresh (1 bunch)
- Bay leaves (2)
- Black pepper
- Cardamom, ground
- Cayenne pepper
- Chinese five-spice powder
- Chives, fresh (1 bunch)
- Cilantro, fresh (1 bunch)
- Cinnamon, ground

- Cloves, ground
- Coriander, ground
- Cumin, ground
- Dill, fresh (1 bunch)
- Fennel powder
- Garlic powder
- Ginger, fresh (2 teaspoons) Ginger, ground
- Green chili powder
- Mustard, ground
- Nutmeg, ground
- Oregano, dried
- Oregano, fresh (1 bunch)
- Paprika, sweet
- Parsley, fresh (1 bunch)
- Peppercorns, black
- Red pepper flakes
- Thyme, dried
- Thyme, fresh (1 bunch)
- Turmeric, ground

Fish and Seafood
- Cod (4 fillets totaling 12 ounces)
- Salmon (4 fillets totaling 12 ounces)
- Shrimp (8 ounces)
- Tuna, yellowfin (4 fillets totaling 12 ounces)

Meat and Poultry
- Beef, ground, 95% lean (1 pound)

- Beef, roast, chuck or rump (1½ pounds, divided into 1 pound and ½ pound)
- Chicken carcass (1)
- Chicken breasts, boneless, skinless (24 ounces, or family pack)
- Chicken thighs, boneless, skinless (11)
- Pork, top loin (4 chops totaling 12 ounces)

Other

- Baking soda substitute, Ener-G (1½ teaspoons) Beef stock (1 cup)
- Bread crumbs
- Bread, Italian (2 slices)
- Bread, white (8 slices)
- Buckwheat, whole (2 tablespoons)
- Bulgur (6 tablespoons)
- Chickpeas, canned (4 ounces)
- Cooking spray
- Cornstarch Couscous (2½ cups plus 6 tablespoons)
- Flour, all-purpose
- Honey
- Jam, strawberry (¼ cup)
- Linguine
- Oil, canola
- Oil, olive
- Penne
- Sugar, brown
- Sugar, granulated
- Tortillas, flour, 6-inch diameter (2)

- Vanilla extract, pure
- Vinegar, apple cider
- Vinegar, balsamic
- Vinegar, white

Week 3 Meal Plan

Monday:
Breakfast: Cheesy Scrambled Eggs with Fresh Herbs
Lunch: Couscous Burgers
Dinner: Indian Chicken Curry (leftover)
Tuesday:
Breakfast: Mixed-Grain Hot Cereal
Lunch: Crab Cakes with Lime Salsa
Dinner: Sweet and Sour Meat Loaf
Wednesday:
Breakfast: Corn Pudding
Lunch: Sweet and Sour Meat Loaf (leftover)
Dinner: Persian Chicken
Thursday:
Breakfast: Cinnamon-Nutmeg Blueberry Muffins
Lunch: Ginger Beef Salad
Dinner: Herb Pesto Tuna
Friday:
Breakfast: Fruit and Cheese Breakfast Wrap
Lunch: Roasted Beef Stew
Dinner: Lemon-Herb Chicken
Saturday:

Breakfast: Curried Egg Pita Pockets

Lunch: Turkey-Bulgur Soup

Dinner: Grilled Steak with Cucumber-Cilantro Salsa

Sunday:

Breakfast: Strawberry–Cream Cheese Stuffed French Toast

Lunch: Egg White Frittata with Penne

Dinner: Baked Cod with Cucumber-Dill Salsa

Suggested Snacks:

- Cinnamon Applesauce, Festive Berry Parfait, Corn Bread (here)
- Tuna salad
- Cucumber sticks
- Mixed berries
- Graham crackers

Week 3 Shopping List

Fruits and Vegetables

- Apples (2)
- Blueberries (8 ounces)
- Cabbage, green, shredded (½ cup) Carrots (2)
- Celery stalks (3)
- Corn, frozen kernels (2 cups)
- Cucumbers, English (2)
- Garlic (14 cloves or 10 teaspoons minced garlic and 2 cloves) Lemons (6)
- Lettuce, leaf, green (1 head) Limes (5)
- Onion, red (1)

- Onions, sweet (2)
- Peppers, bell, red (3)
- Scallions (4)
- Watercress (1 bunch)

Dairy and Dairy Alternatives

- Butter, unsalted (¾ cup)
- Cheese, cream, plain (10 ounces) Eggs (24)
- Milk, coconut (¼ cup)
- Milk, rice, unsweetened (4 cups)
- Milk, rice, vanilla (1¼ cups)
- Sour cream, light
- (4 tablespoons)

Spices and Herbs

- Basil, fresh (1 bunch)
- Bay leaves, dried (2)
- Cayenne pepper
- Chives, fresh (1 bunch)
- Cilantro, fresh (1 bunch)
- Cinnamon, ground
- Cumin, ground
- Curry powder
- Dill, fresh (1 bunch)
- Garlic powder
- Ginger, fresh (4-inch piece) Ginger, ground
- Green chili powder
- Nutmeg, ground
- Oregano, dried

- Oregano, fresh (1 bunch)
- Paprika, sweet
- Parsley, fresh (1 bunch)
- Peppercorns, black, freshly ground Red pepper flakes
- Sage, fresh (1 bunch)
- Tarragon, fresh (1 bunch)
- Thyme, fresh (1 bunch)

Fish and Seafood

- Cod (4 fillets totaling 12 ounces)
- Crab meat, queen (8 ounces)
- Tuna, yellowfin (4 fillets totaling 12 ounces)

Meat and Poultry

- Beef, ground, 95% lean (1 pound)
- Beef, roast, chuck (½ pound)
- Beef, steak, flank (¾ pound)
- Beef, tenderloin (4 steaks totaling 12 ounces)
- Chicken breasts, boneless, skinless (12 ounces)
- Chicken thighs, boneless, skinless (11)
- Pork, top loin (4 chops totaling 12 ounces)
- Turkey, ground, 93% lean (5 ounces)

Other

- Baking soda substitute, Ener-G (3½ teaspoons)
- Bread crumbs
- Bread, pita pockets, 4-inch diameter (2)
- Bread, white (8 slices)
- Buckwheat, whole (2 tablespoons)
- Bulgur (1 cup)
- Chickpeas (4 ounces)

- Chili paste (1 teaspoon)
- Cooking spray
- Cornstarch
- Couscous (3 cups)
- Flour, all-purpose
- Honey
- Hot pepper sauce
- Jam, strawberry (¼ cup)
- Oil, canola
- Oil, olive
- Penne
- Stock, beef (1 cup)
- Sugar, brown
- Sugar, granulated
- Tortillas, flour, 6-inch diameter (2)
- Vanilla extract, pure
- Rinegar, Apple cader
- Vinegar, white

Week 4 Meal Plan

Monday:
Breakfast: Egg-in-the-Hole
Lunch: Crab Cakes with Lime Salsa
Dinner: Pesto Pork Chops
Tuesday:
Breakfast: Corn Pudding
Lunch: Five-Spice Chicken Lettuce Wraps

Dinner: Sweet Glazed Salmon

Wednesday:

Breakfast: Fruit and Cheese Breakfast Wrap

Lunch: Egg White Frittata with Penne

Dinner: Indian Chicken Curry

Thursday:

Breakfast: Rhubarb Bread Pudding

Lunch: Indian Chicken Curry

Dinner: Couscous Burgers

Friday:

Breakfast: Mixed-Grain Hot Cereal

Lunch: Traditional Chicken-Vegetable Soup

Dinner: Grilled Steak with Cucumber-Cilantro Salsa

Saturday:

Breakfast: Skillet-Baked Pancake

Lunch: Linguine with Roasted Red Pepper–Basil Sauce

Dinner: Herb Pesto Tuna

Sunday:

Breakfast: Cheesy Scrambled Eggs with Fresh Herbs

Lunch: Roasted Beef Stew

Dinner: Lemon-Herb Chicken

Suggested Snacks:

- Cinnamon Applesauce, Blueberry-Pineapple Smoothie, Roasted Red
- Pepper and Chicken Crostini, Deviled eggs
- Grapes
- Vanilla wafer cookies
- Carrot sticks

Week 4 Shopping List

Fruits and Vegetables

- Apples (2)
- Carrots (2)
- Celery stalks (4)
- Corn, frozen kernels (2 cups)
- Cucumber, English (1)
- Garlic (14 cloves or 10 teaspoons minced garlic and 2 cloves)
- Lemons (4)
- Lettuce, Boston (1 head)
- Limes (3)
- Onions, sweet (4)
- Peppers, red, bell (2)
- Rhubarb (6 stalks)
- Scallions (4)
- Sprouts, bean (½ cup)

Dairy and Dairy Alternatives

- Butter, unsalted (¾ cup)
- Cheese, cream, plain (5 ounces)
- Cheese, Parmesan, low-fat (1 ounce) Eggs (25)
- Milk, coconut (¼ cup)
- Milk, rice, unsweetened (3¼ cups)
- Milk, rice, vanilla (1¼ cups)
- Sour cream, light (2 tablespoons)

Spices and Herbs

- Basil, fresh (1 bunch)

- Cayenne pepper
- Chinese five-spice powder
- Chives, fresh (1 bunch)
- Cilantro, fresh (1 bunch)
- Cinnamon, ground
- Curry powder
- Ginger, fresh (2-inch piece)
- Green chili powder
- Nutmeg, ground
- Oregano, fresh (1 bunch)
- Parsley, fresh (1 bunch)
- Pepper, black, freshly ground
- Red pepper flakes
- Tarragon, fresh (1 bunch)
- Thyme, fresh (1 bunch)
- Vanilla bean (1)

Fish and Seafood

- Crab meat, queen (8 ounces)
- Salmon (4 fillets totaling 12 ounces) Tuna,
- yellowfin (4 fillets totaling 12 ounces)

Meat and Poultry

- Beef, roast, chuck (½ pound)
- Beef, tenderloin (4 steaks totaling 12 ounces)
- Chicken breasts, boneless, skinless (32 ounces, or family pack)
- Chicken thighs, boneless, skinless (6)
- Pork, chops, top loin (4 chops totaling 12 ounces)

Other

- Baking soda substitute, Ener-G (½ teaspoon)
- Bread crumbs
- Bread, Italian (1 loaf)
- Bread, white (10 slices)
- Buckwheat, whole (2 tablespoons)
- Bulgur (6 tablespoons)
- Chickpeas (4 ounces)
- Cooking spray
- Cornstarch
- Couscous (2 cups)
- Flour, all-purpose
- Honey
- Hot pepper sauce
- Oil, olive
- Penne
- Spaghetti
- Stock, beef (1 cup)
- Sugar, granulated
- 6-inch diameter
- Tortillas, flour, (2)
- Vinegar,balsamic.

Chapter 6: Recipes of Kitchen Staples

This chapter comprises of the kitchen staple recipes that need to be kept in store while following a renal diet.

6.1. Balsamic Vinaigrette

(Serving: 1, Cook Time: 5 Minutes, Difficulty: Easy)

Ingredients:

- 1½ cups extra virgin olive oil
- 1 cup good-quality balsamic vinegar
- 2 tablespoons chopped fresh parsley
- 2 tablespoons minced onion
- 1 teaspoon minced garlic
- 4 teaspoons chopped fresh basil
- Freshly ground black pepper

Instructions:

1. Whisk together the olive oil and balsamic vinegar in a large bowl for about 1 minute before the ingredients are emulsified. Apply the parsley, cabbage, garlic, and basil to the whisk. And spice seasoning.

2. Move the vinaigrette to a glass jar with a lid and prepare it for up to 2 weeks at room temperature. Until using, shake.

6.2. Homemade Mayonnaise

(Serving: 1, Cook Time: 10 Minutes, Difficulty: Easy)

Ingredients:

- 2 egg yolks, at room temperature

- 1½ teaspoons freshly squeezed lemon juice
- ¼ teaspoon mustard powder
- ¾ cup olive oil

Instructions:

1. Whisk the yolks, lemon juice, and mustard together in a medium bowl for about 30 seconds or until well mixed. In a small, steady stream, apply the olive oil while whisking for about 3 minutes or until the oil is emulsified and the mayonnaise is thick. Place the mayonnaise in a sealed tub for up to 1 week in the refrigerator.

6.3. Balsamic Reduction

(Serving: 1, Cook Time: 30 Minutes, Difficulty: Normal)

Ingredients:

- 2 cups good-quality
- balsamic vinegar
- 1 tablespoon granulated sugar

Instructions:

1. Over a medium-high fire, put a small saucepan and whisk together the balsamic vinegar and sugar. Put it to a boil with the vinegar mixture.

2. Reduce the heat to low and boil, stirring regularly, until the vinegar is reduced or for about 20 minutes. Remove the reduction in the vinegar from the heat and allow it to cool completely. Move the refrigerated reduction to a freezer and store it for up to 2 weeks at room temperature.

6.4. Herb Pesto

(Serving: 1, Cook Time: 10 Minutes, Difficulty: Easy)

Ingredient:

- 1 cup packed fresh basil leaves
- ½ cup packed fresh oregano leaves
- ½ cup packed fresh parsley leaves
- 2 garlic cloves ¼ cup olive oil
- 2 tablespoons freshly squeezed lemon juice

Instructions:

1. In a food processor, put the basil, oregano, parsley, and garlic and pulse for around 3 minutes or until very finely chopped. Drizzle the pesto with the olive oil until a thick paste develops, rubbing the sides down at least once.

2. Apply the juice and pump of the lemon until well combined. Place the pesto for up to 1 week in the refrigerator in a sealed jar.

6.5. Alfredo Sauce

(Serving: 8, Cook Time: 10 Minutes, Difficulty: Normal)

Ingredients:

- 2 tablespoons unsalted butter
- 1½ tablespoons all-purpose flour
- 1 teaspoon minced garlic
- 1 cup plain unsweetened rice milk
- ¾ cup plain cream cheese
- 2 tablespoons Parmesan cheese

- ¼ teaspoon ground nutmeg
- Freshly ground black pepper, for seasoning

Instructions:

1. Melt the butter in a medium saucepan over medium heat. To form a paste, whisk in the flour and garlic and continue whisking for 2 minutes to cook the flour. In the rice milk, whisk and whisk for about 4 minutes or until the mixture is nearly thick and boiling. Whisk in the cream cheese, nutmeg, and parmesan cheese for around 1 minute or until the sauce is tender. From the heat, extract the sauce and season with pepper.

2. Serve over spaghetti immediately.

6.6. Apple-Cranberry Chutney

(Serving: 1, Cook Time: 30 Minutes, Difficulty: Normal)

Instructions:

- 1 large apple, peeled, cored, and sliced thin
- ½ cup granulated sugar
- ½ cup fresh cranberries
- ½ red onion, finely chopped
- ¼ cup apple juice
- ¼ cup apple cider vinegar
- Freshly ground black pepper, for seasoning

Instructions:

1. In a medium saucepan over medium heat, stir together the apple, sugar, cranberries, onion, apple juice, and vinegar. Bring the mixture to a boil, and then reduce the heat to low and cook, frequently stirring, for 25 to 30 minutes or until the cranberries are very tender.

2. Season with pepper. Remove the chutney from the heat and chill in the refrigerator for about 3 hours or completely cool.

3. Store the chutney in a sealed container in the refrigerator for up to 1 week.

6.7. Cooked Four-Pepper Salsa

(Serving: 1, Cook Time: 1 Hours 10 Minutes, Difficulty: Normal)

Ingredients:

- 1-pound red bell peppers, boiled and chopped
- 2 small sweet banana peppers, chopped
- 1 small sweet onion, chopped
- 1 jalapeño pepper, finely chopped
- 1 green bell pepper, chopped
- ½ cup apple cider vinegar
- 2 teaspoons minced garlic
- 1 tablespoon granulated sugar
- 3 tablespoons chopped fresh cilantro

Instructions:

1. Mix the red bell peppers, banana peppers, tomato, jalapeño pepper, green bell pepper, apple cider vinegar, garlic, and sugar in a big saucepan over medium heat. Get the mixture, constantly stirring, to a boil.

2. Reduce the heat to low and simmer, constantly stirring, for around 1 hour. Stir in the

cilantro and cook for 15 minutes, stirring regularly.

3. Take the salsa out of the sun and let it cool for 15 to 20 minutes. Move the salsa to a refrigerator and chill in the fridge for up to 1 week before you can use it. Serve cold with fried tortilla chips.

6.8. Easy Chicken Stock

(Serving: 1, Cook Time: 7 to 8 hours, Difficulty: Hard)

Ingredients:

- 1 roasted chicken carcass, skin removed
- Water
- 1 tablespoon apple cider vinegar
- 4 celery stalks, chopped into
- 2-inch pieces
- 2 sweet onions, peeled and quartered
- 2 carrots, cut into
- 2-inch chunks
- 2 garlic cloves, crushed
- 2 bay leaves
- 5 fresh thyme sprigs
- 5 fresh parsley stems
- ½ teaspoon black peppercorns

Instructions:

1. In a big 4-to 6-quart stockpot, place the chicken carcass, breaking it into smaller parts to make it fit, if appropriate. Cover the carcass with water and apply the apple cider vinegar until the liquid fills the carcass by around 1 inch. Place the stockpot until the liquid simmers over medium heat and then reduce the heat to mild to simmer very

gently. For 5 or 6 hours, boil the carcass, adding more water if the top of the carcass is uncovered. On the stock, skim off any accumulated foam. To the stockpot, add the celery, cabbage, carrots, garlic, bay leaves, thyme, parsley, and peppercorns.

2. Simmer for 2 hours, adding more water to keep the ingredients covered, if possible. Strain the stock and discard the solids using a fine-mesh strainer. Let the stock cool and store it in the refrigerator for up to 1 week or up to 6 months in the freezer.

3. Dialysis modification: To raise the volume and decrease potassium, add water when the stock is finished. The chicken taste would not be so diluted by as much as 3 or 4 cups of water, so make sure to taste as you add water to achieve an appropriate flavor.

6.9. Cinnamon Applesauce

(Serving: 1, Cook Time: 30 Minutes, Difficulty: Normal)

Ingredients:

- 8 apples, peeled, cored, and sliced thin
- ½ cup water
- 1 teaspoon ground cinnamon
- ¼ teaspoon ground nutmeg
- Pinch ground allspice

Instructions:

1. Place the apples, water, cinnamon, nutmeg, and allspice over medium heat in a medium saucepan. Heat the mixture of apples, stirring regularly, for 25 to 30 minutes, or until the apples are tender. To mash the apples to the perfect texture, remove the saucepan from the heat and use a potato masher.

2. Let cool the applesauce for up to 1 week of storage in the refrigerator.

6.10. Lemon Curd

(Serving: 1, Cook Time: 10 Minutes, Difficulty: Normal)

Ingredients:

- 6 large egg yolks
- ¾ cup granulated sugar
- Zest of 4 lemons
- Juice of 4 lemons
- ½ cup unsalted butter, cut into 1-inch pieces

Instructions:

1. In a small saucepan, pour about 2 inches of water and put over medium heat until the water simmers. The water softly simmers, reduce the heat to low, and place a medium stainless-steel bowl over the saucepan. Whisk the egg yolks, sugar, lemon zest, and lemon juice together in the bowl for 8 to 10 minutes or until the mixture forms thick ribbons when the whisk is removed. Remove the saucepan from the bowl and whisk in the cubes of butter, one at a time, until each is thoroughly combined well. Onto another medium cup, drain the lemon curd through a fine-mesh strainer. To press through additional curd, and squeeze out the zest, use the back of a spoon.

2. In the strainer, discard the zest and cover the lemon curd with plastic wrap, pressed straight onto the card base. For around 3 hours or until set, chill in the refrigerator.

Store in the refrigerator in a sealed container for up to 1 week.

6.11. Traditional Beef Stock

(Serving: 1, Cook Time: 13 Hours, Difficulty: Normal)

Ingredients:

- 2 pounds beef bones (beef marrow, knuckle bones, or ribs)
- 1 celery stalk, chopped into 2-inch pieces
- 1 carrot, peeled and roughly chopped

- ½ sweet onion, peeled and quartered
- 3 garlic cloves, crushed
- 1 teaspoon black peppercorns
- 3 sprigs thyme
- 2 bay leaves
- Water

Instructions:

1. Preheat the oven to about 350°F. Put the bones in a deep baking pan and roast them in the oven for 30 minutes, rotating once. Move the roasted bones to a large stockpot and add about 3 inches of celery, carrots, onion, garlic, peppercorns, thyme, bay leaves, and ample water to cover the bones.

2. Lower the heat and simmer the stock for at least 12 hours. During the first 4 hours, inspect the broth every hour to skim off any foam or impurities from the surface. Remove the pot from the heat and refrigerate for 30 minutes. Using tongs, remove the broad bones, strain the stock through a fine-mesh strainer, and put the strainer's strong parts. In jars or pots, pour the stock and allow it to cool fully.

3. Hold the beef stock for up to 6 days in packed containers or cans in the refrigerator or 3-months in the freezer.

Chapter 7: Spice Blends and Seasonings

Renal patients can follow a health instilling diet besides treating their taste buds well with these flavorsome spice blends and seasonings.

7.1. Fajita Rub

(Serving: 1, Cook Time: 5 Minutes, Difficulty: Easy)

Ingredients:

- 1½ teaspoons chili powder
- 1 teaspoon garlic powder
- 1 teaspoon roasted cumin seed
- 1 teaspoon dried oregano
- ½ teaspoon ground coriander
- ¼ teaspoon red pepper flakes

Instructions:

1. In a blender, place the chili powder, garlic powder, cumin seed, oregano, coriander, and red pepper flakes, and pulse until the ingredients are well mixed and ground.

2. To a small jar with a lid, move the spice mixture. Up to 6 months of storage in a cold,

dry location.

7.2. Dried Herb Rub

(Serving: 1, Cook Time: 5 Minutes, Difficulty: Easy)

Ingredients:

- 1 tablespoon dried thyme
- 1 tablespoon dried oregano

- 1 tablespoon dried parsley
- 2 teaspoons dried basil
- 2 teaspoons ground coriander
- 2 teaspoons onion powder
- 1 teaspoon ground cumin
- 1 teaspoon garlic powder
- 1 teaspoon paprika
- ½ teaspoon cayenne pepper

Instructions:

1. In a blender, add thyme, oregano, parsley, basil, cilantro, onion powder, cumin, garlic powder, paprika, and cayenne pepper pulse until the ingredients are soft and well mixed. Move the rub to a small, lid-based jar.

2. Up to 6 months of storage in a cold, dry location.

7.3. Mediterranean Seasoning

(Serving: 1, Cook Time: 5 Minutes, Difficulty: Easy)

Ingredients:

- 2 tablespoons dried oregano
- 1 tablespoon dried thyme
- 2 teaspoons dried rosemary, chopped finely or crushed
- 2 teaspoons dried basil
- 1 teaspoon dried marjoram
- 1 teaspoon dried parsley flakes

Instructions:

1. Mix the oregano, thyme, rosemary, basil, marjoram, and parsley in a small bowl until well mixed. To a small jar with a lid, move the seasoning mixture.

2. Store in a cool, dry place for up to 6 months.

7.4. Hot Curry Powder

(Serving: 1, Cook Time: 5 Minutes, Difficulty: Easy)
Ingredients:

- ¼ cup ground cumin
- ¼ cup ground coriander
- 3 tablespoons turmeric
- 2 tablespoons sweet paprika
- 2 tablespoons ground mustard
- 1 tablespoon fennel powder
- ½ teaspoon green chili powder
- 2 teaspoons ground cardamom
- 1 teaspoon ground cinnamon
- ½ teaspoon ground cloves

Instructions:

1. Put the cumin, coriander, turmeric, paprika, mustard, fennel powder, green chili powder, cardamom, cinnamon, cloves into a blender, and pulse until the ingredients are

ground and well combined. Transfer the curry powder to a small container with a lid. Store in a cool, dry place for up to 6 months. Dialysis modification: 2. Omit the sweet paprika to reduce the amount of potassium. It will change the curry powder's color, but the other spices have a strong enough flavor to make up for the omission.

7.5. Cajun Seasoning

(Serving: 1, Cook Time: 5 Minutes, Difficulty: Easy)

Ingredients:

- ½ cup sweet paprika
- ¼ cup garlic powder
- 3 tablespoons onion powder
- 3 tablespoons freshly ground black pepper
- 2 tablespoons dried oregano
- 1 tablespoon cayenne pepper
- 1 tablespoon dried thyme

Instructions:

1. In a blender, place the paprika, garlic powder, onion powder, black pepper, oregano, cayenne pepper, and thyme, and process until the ingredients are well mixed and ground. To a small jar with a lid, move the seasoning mixture.

2. Store for up to 6 months in a cold, dry location.

7.6. Apple Pie Spice

(Serving: 1, Cook Time: 5 Minutes, Difficulty: Easy)

Ingredients:

- ¼ cup ground cinnamon
- 2 teaspoons ground nutmeg
- 2 teaspoons ground ginger
- 1 teaspoon allspice
- ½ teaspoon ground cloves

Instructions:

1. Mix the cinnamon, nutmeg, ginger, allspice, and cloves in a small bowl until the spices are well mixed. To a small jar with a lid, move the spice mixture.

2. Up to 6 months of storage in a cold, dry location.

7.7. Ras El Hanout

(Serving: 1, Cook Time: 5 Minutes, Difficulty: Easy)

Ingredients:

- 2 teaspoons ground nutmeg
- 2 teaspoons ground coriander
- 2 teaspoons ground cumin
- 2 teaspoons turmeric
- 2 teaspoons cinnamon
- 1 teaspoon cardamom
- 1 teaspoon sweet paprika
- 1 teaspoon ground mace
- 1 teaspoon freshly ground black pepper
- 1 teaspoon cayenne pepper
- ½ teaspoon ground allspice
- ½ teaspoon ground cloves

Instructions:

1. Add nutmeg, cilantro, cumin, turmeric, cinnamon, cardamom, paprika, mace, black

pepper, cayenne pepper, allspice, and cloves together in a small bowl until the spices are well mixed. To a small jar with a lid, move the seasoning mixture.

2. Store in a cool, dry place for up to 6 months.

7.8. Poultry Seasoning

(Serving: 1, Cook Time: 5 Minutes, Difficulty: Easy)

Ingredients:

- 2 tablespoons ground thyme

- 2 tablespoons ground marjoram
- 1 tablespoon ground sage
- 1 tablespoon ground celery seed
- 1 teaspoon ground rosemary
- 1 teaspoon freshly ground black pepper

Instructions:

1. Mix the thyme, marjoram, sage, celery seed, rosemary, and pepper together in a small bowl until the spices are well mixed. To a small jar with a lid, move the seasoning mixture.

2. Store in a cool, dry place for up to 6 months.

7.9. Berbere SPICE MIX

(Serving: 1, Cook Time: 5 Minutes, Difficulty: Easy)

Ingredients:

- 1 tablespoon coriander seeds
- 1 teaspoon cumin seeds
- 1 teaspoon fenugreek seeds
- ¼ teaspoon black peppercorns
- ¼ teaspoon whole allspice berries
- 4 whole cloves
- 4 dried chiles, stemmed and seeded
- ¼ cup dried onion flakes
- 2 tablespoons ground cardamom
- 1 tablespoon sweet paprika
- 1 teaspoon ground ginger
- ½ teaspoon ground nutmeg
- ½ teaspoon ground cinnamon

Instructions:

1. Mix the thyme, marjoram, sage, celery seed, rosemary, and pepper together in a small bowl until the spices are well mixed. To a small jar with a lid, move the seasoning mixture.

7.10. Creole Seasoning Mix

(Serving: 1, Cook Time: 5 Minutes, Difficulty: Easy)

Ingredients:

- 1 tablespoon sweet paprika
- 1 tablespoon garlic powder
- 2 teaspoons onion powder
- 2 teaspoons dried oregano
- 1 teaspoon cayenne pepper
- 1 teaspoon ground thyme
- 1 teaspoon freshly ground black pepper

Instructions:

1. In a small container, mix together the, onion powder, oregano, paprika, garlic powder, cayenne pepper, thyme, and black pepper until the ingredients are well combined. To

a small jar with a lid, move the seasoning mixture.

2. Store in a cool, dry place for up to 6 months.

7.11. Adobo Seasoning Mix

(Serving: 2, Cook Time: 30 Minutes, Difficulty: Normal)

Ingredients:

- 4 tablespoons garlic powder
- 4 tablespoons onion powder

- 4 tablespoons ground cumin
- 3 tablespoons dried oregano
- 3 tablespoons freshly ground black pepper
- 2 tablespoons sweet paprika
- 2 tablespoons ground chili powder
- 1 tablespoon ground turmeric
- 1 tablespoon ground coriander

Instructions:

1. In a small bowl, mix together the oregano, black pepper, paprika, chili powder, garlic powder, onion powder, cumin, turmeric, and coriander until the ingredients are well combined.

2. Shift the seasoning mix to a small jar with a lid and store in a cool, dry place for up to 6 months.

7.12. Herbes De Provence

(Serving: 1, Cook Time: 5 Minutes, Difficulty: Easy)

Ingredients:

- ½ cup dried thyme
- 3 tablespoons dried marjoram
- 3 tablespoons dried savory
- 2 tablespoons dried rosemary
- 2 teaspoons dried lavender flowers
- 1 teaspoon ground fennel

Instructions

1. Put the thyme, marjoram, savory, rosemary, lavender, and fennel in a blender and pulse a few times to amalgamate. Shift the herb mix to a small jar with a lid.

2. Store for up to 6 months in a dry and cold location.

7.13. Lamb and Pork Seasoning

(Serving: 1, Cook Time: 5 Minutes, Difficulty: Easy)

Ingredients:

- ¼ cup celery seed
- 2 tablespoons dried oregano
- 2 tablespoons onion powder
- 1 tablespoon dried thyme
- 1½ teaspoons garlic powder
- 1 teaspoon crushed bay leaf
- 1 teaspoon freshly ground black pepper
- 1 teaspoon ground allspice

Instructions:

1. Put the celery seed, bay leaf, pepper, oregano, onion powder, thyme, garlic powder, and allspice in a blender and pulse a few times to combine.

2. Shift the herb mixture to a small jar with a lid. Up to 6 months, store in a cold, dry location.

7.14. Asian Seasoning

(Serving: 1, Cook Time: 5 Minutes, Difficulty: Easy)

Ingredients:

- 2 tablespoons sesame seeds
- 2 tablespoons onion powder
- 2 tablespoons crushed star anise pods
- 2 tablespoons ground ginger

- 1 teaspoon ground allspice
- ½ teaspoon cardamom
- ½ teaspoon ground cloves

Instructions

1. In a small bowl, mix the sesame seeds, onion powder, star anise, ginger, allspice, cardamom, and cloves until well combined.

2.Transfer the spice mixture to a small container with a lid. Store in a cool, dry place for up to 6 months.

7.15. Onion Seasoning Blend

(Serving: 1, Cook Time: 5 Minutes, Difficulty: Easy)

Ingredients:

- 2 tablespoons onion powder
- 1 tablespoon dry mustard
- 2 teaspoons sweet paprika
- 2 teaspoons garlic powder
- 1 teaspoon dried thyme
- ½ teaspoon celery seeds
- ½ teaspoon freshly ground black pepper

Instructions:

1. In a small bowl, mix the celery seeds, onion powder, mustard, paprika, garlic powder, thyme, and pepper until well combined.

2. To a small jar with a lid, move the spice mixture. Up to 6 months of storage in a cold, dry location.

7.16. Coffee Dry Rub

(Serving: 1, Cook Time: 5 Minutes, Difficulty: Easy)

Ingredients:

- 1 tablespoon ground coffee
- 2 teaspoons ground cumin
- 2 teaspoons sweet paprika
- 2 teaspoons chili powder
- 1 teaspoon brown sugar
- ¼ teaspoon freshly ground black pepper

Instructions:

1. In a small bowl, mix the brown sugar, coffee, cumin, paprika, chili powder, and pepper until well combined. Move the rub to a small, lid-based jar.

2. Up to 6 months, store in a cold, dry location.

Chapter 8: Dessert and Smoothie Recipes

This chapter has a range of dessert recipes that can be cooked while following a renal diet.

8.1. Apple-Chai Smoothie

(Serving: 2, Cook Time: 35 Minutes, Difficulty: Normal)

Ingredients:

- 1 cup unsweetened rice milk
- 1 chai tea bag
- 1 apple, peeled, cored, and chopped
- 2 cups ice

Instructions:

1. Heat the rice milk in a medium saucepan over low heat for about 5 minutes or until steaming.

2. Remove the milk from the heat and steeply add the teabag. Let the milk cool for about 30 minutes in the refrigerator with the tea bag, remove the teabag, and squeeze gently to release all the flavor.

3. In a blender, put the milk, apple, and ice and blend until smooth. Pour 2-glasses into them and serve.

8.2. Watermelon-Raspberry Smoothie

(Serving: 2, Cook Time: 10 Minutes, Difficulty: Easy)

Ingredients:

- ½ cup boiled, cooled, and shredded red cabbage
- 1 cup diced watermelon
- ½ cup fresh raspberries

- 1 cup ice

Instructions:

1. In a blender, put the cabbage and pump for 2 minutes or until it is finely chopped.

2. Attach the watermelon and raspberries and pulse until very well mixed, or around 2-minute.

3. Until the smoothie is very rich and smooth, apply the ice and mix. Pour two glasses into them and serve.

8.3. Festive Berry Parfait

(Serving: 4, Cook Time: 1 hour 20 Minutes, Difficulty: Normal)

Ingredients:

- 1 cup vanilla rice milk, at room temperature
- ½ cup plain cream cheese, at room temperature
- 1 tablespoon granulated sugar
- ½ teaspoon ground cinnamon
- 1 cup crumbled Meringue Cookies (here)
- 2 cups fresh blueberries
- 1 cup sliced fresh strawberries

Instructions:

1. Whisk the milk, cream cheese, sugar, and cinnamon together in a small cup until smooth. Spoon 1/4 cup of the crumbled cookie into 4 (6-ounce) glasses at the bottom of each.

2. On top of the cakes, spoon 1/4 cup of the cream cheese mixture. Place 1/4 cup of the berries on top of the cream cheese. Repeat with the cookies, cream cheese mixture, and berries in each cup.

3. For 1 hour, cool in the refrigerator and serve.

8.4. Mixed-Grain Hot Cereal

(Serving: 4, Cook Time: 35 Minutes, Difficulty: Normal)

Ingredients:

- 2¼ cups water
- 1¼ cups vanilla rice milk
- 6 tablespoons uncooked bulgur
- 2 tablespoons uncooked whole buckwheat
- 1 cup peeled, sliced apple
- 6 tablespoons plain uncooked couscous
- ½ teaspoon ground cinnamon

Instructions:

1. Heat the water and milk in a medium saucepan over medium-high heat. Bring the bulgur, buckwheat, and apple to a boil, and add them.

2. Reduce the heat to low and simmer, stirring regularly, until the bulgur is tender or for

20 to 25 minutes.

3. Stir in the couscous and cinnamon and remove the saucepan from the sun.

For 10 minutes, let the saucepan rest, sealed, then fluff the cereal with a fork before eating.

8.5. Blueberry-Pineapple Smoothie

(Serving: 2, Cook Time: 15 Minutes, Difficulty: Easy)

Ingredients:

- 1 cup frozen blueberries
- ½ cup pineapple chunks
- ½ cup English cucumber

- ½ apple ½ cup water

Instructions:

1. In a blender, put the blueberries, pineapple, cucumber, apple, and water and combine until thick and creamy. Pour 2 glasses into them and serve.

8.6. Corn Pudding

(Serving: 6, Cook Time: 50 Minutes, Difficulty: Normal)

Ingredients:

- Unsalted butter, for greasing the baking dish
- 2 tablespoons all-purpose flour
- ½ teaspoon Ener-G baking soda substitute
- 3 eggs
- ¾ cup unsweetened rice milk, at room temperature
- 3 tablespoons unsalted butter, melted
- 2 tablespoons light sour cream
- 2 tablespoons granulated sugar
- 2 cups frozen corn kernels, thawed

Instructions:

1. Preheat the oven to about 350°F. Lightly oil a buttery, 8-by-8-inch baking dish; set aside. Stir the flour and baking soda replacement together in a shallow bowl; set aside.

2. Whisk the eggs, rice milk, butter, sour cream, and sugar together in a medium dish.

Stir the flour mixture, when smooth, into the egg mixture.

3. Apply the corn to the batter and stir until it is combined very well. Into the baking bowl, spoon the batter, and bake for about 40 minutes or until the pudding is set. Let the pudding cool for 15 minutes or so and serve until soft.

8.7. Rhubarb Bread Pudding

(Serving: 6, Cook Time: 1 Hour 30 Minutes, Difficulty: Easy)

Ingredients:

- Unsalted butter, for greasing the baking dish
- 1½ cups unsweetened rice milk
- 3 eggs
- ½ cup granulated sugar
- 1 tablespoon cornstarch
- 1 vanilla bean, split
- 10 thick pieces white bread, cut into 1-inch chunks
- 2 cups chopped fresh rhubarb

Instructions:

1. Preheat the oven to about 350°F. Lightly oil a buttery, 8-by-8-inch baking dish; set aside. Whisk the rice milk, eggs, sugar, and cornstarch together in a large dish. In the milk mixture, scrape the vanilla seeds and whisk to combine.

2. Apply the egg mixture to the bread and whisk to cover the bread fully. To mix, add the chopped rhubarb and stir. Leave the mixture of bread and egg to soak for 30 minutes. In

the prepared baking dish, spoon the mixture, cover it with aluminum foil and bake for 40 minutes. Uncover and bake the bread pudding for an extra 10 minutes or until the pudding is brown and set. Serve it sweet.

3. Dialysis modification: To get the potassium to less than 150 mg per serving, reduce the rhubarb to 1 cup. Or omit the rhubarb to get the potassium down to less than 75 mg per serving. The pudding for bread is

Yummy without rhubarb, so it's going to be less tart.

8.8. Cinnamon-Nutmeg Blueberry Muffins

(Serving: 12, Cook Time: 45 Minutes, Difficulty: Normal)

Ingredients:

- 2 cups unsweetened rice milk
- 1 tablespoon apple cider vinegar
- 3½ cups all-purpose flour
- 1 cup granulated sugar
- 1 tablespoon Ener-G baking soda substitute
- 1 teaspoon ground cinnamon
- ½ teaspoon ground nutmeg
- Pinch ground ginger
- ½ cup canola oil
- 2 tablespoons pure vanilla extract
- 2½ cups fresh blueberries

Instructions:

1. Preheat the oven to about 375°F. Cover the cups with paper liners from a muffin pan; set aside. Stir together the rice milk and the vinegar in a small bowl; set aside for 10 minutes. Stir the flour, sugar, baking soda replacement, cinnamon, nutmeg, and ginger

together in a wide bowl until well combined.

2. To mix the milk mixture, add the oil and vanilla and whisk to combine. To the dry ingredients, add the milk mixture and stir until just mixed. Fold the blueberries in it. Spoon uniformly into the cups with the muffin batter.

3. Cook the muffins for 25 to 30 minutes or until the muffins are golden, and a toothpick inserted in the middle comes out clean. Enable the muffins to cool before serving for 15 minutes.

8.9. Fruit and Cheese Wrap

(Serving: 2, Cook Time: 10 Minutes, Difficulty: Easy)

Ingredients:

- 2 (6-inch) flour tortillas
- 2 tablespoons plain cream cheese
- 1 apple, peeled, cored, and sliced thin
- 1 tablespoon honey

Instructions:

1. On a clean working surface, lay all tortillas and sprinkle 1-tablespoon of cream cheese on each tortilla, leaving around 1/2 inch around the edges.

2. On the cream cheese, just off the middle of the tortilla on the side nearest to you, place the apple slices, leaving about 1 1/2 inches on either side and 2 inches on the rim.

3. Drizzle gently with honey on the apples. Fold the tortillas' left and right sides to the middle, laying the side over the apples.

4. Fold it over the fruit and the side bits by choosing the tortilla edge nearest to you. Roll the tortilla to create a snug wrap away from you. With the second tortilla, refresh.

8.10. Strawberry–Cream Cheese Stuffed French Toast

(Serving: 4, Cook Time: 1 Hour 5 Minutes, Difficulty: Normal)

Ingredients:

- Cooking spray, for greasing the baking dish
- ½ cup plain cream cheese
- 4 tablespoons strawberry jam
- 8 slices thick white bread
- 2 eggs, beaten

- ½ cup unsweetened rice milk
- 1 teaspoon pure vanilla extract
- 1 tablespoon granulated sugar
- ¼ teaspoon ground cinnamon

Instructions:

1. Preheat the oven to about 350°F. Use cooking spray to spray an 8-by-8-inch baking dish; set aside. Stir the cream cheese and the jam together in a small bowl until well blended.

2. To make sandwiches, spread 3-tablespoons of the cream cheese mixture on 4-slices of bread and top with the remaining 4-slices. Whisk the eggs, milk, and vanilla in a medium bowl until smooth.

3. In the egg mixture, dip the sandwiches and lay them in the baking dish. Over the sandwiches, pour any leftover egg mixture and sprinkle them with sugar and cinnamon equally.

4. Cover the dish and refrigerate overnight with foil. Bake the covered French toast for 1 hour. Remove the foil and cook for more than 5 minutes or until the French toast is golden. Serve it sweet.

Chapter 9: Snack Recipes

In this chapter, we have compiled an amazingly delicious range of snack recipes for renal patients.

9.1. Roasted Onion Garlic Dip

(Serving: 1, Cook Time: 1 Hour, Difficulty: Normal)

Ingredients:

- 1 large sweet onion, peeled and cut into eighths
- 8 garlic cloves
- 2 teaspoons olive oil
- ½ cup light sour cream
- 1 tablespoon fresh lemon juice
- 1 tablespoon chopped fresh parsley
- 1 teaspoon chopped fresh thyme
- Freshly ground black pepper

Instructions:

1. Preheat the oven to about 425 °F. Toss the onion and garlic with the olive oil in a shallow cup. To a piece of aluminum foil, move the onion and garlic and loosely bundle the vegetables in a packet. Place a small baking sheet with the foil packet and place the sheet in the oven. Roast the vegetables, or until they are very fragrant and yellow, for 50 minutes to 1 hour. Take the packet out of the oven and let it cool for 15 minutes.

2. Stir the sour cream, lemon juice, parsley, thyme, and black pepper together in a medium dish. Carefully open the foil package and pass the vegetables onto a cutting board. Chop the vegetables and add them to the mixture with sour cream. Stir to blend.

9.2. Baba Ghanoush

(Serving: 6, Cook Time: 30 Minutes, Difficulty: Normal)

Ingredients:

- 1 medium eggplant, halved and scored with a crosshatch pattern on the cut sides
- 1 tablespoon olive oil, plus extra for brushing
- 1 large sweet onion, peeled and diced
- 2 garlic cloves, halved
- 1 teaspoon ground cumin
- 1 teaspoon ground coriander
- 1 tablespoon lemon juice
- Freshly ground black pepper

Instructions:

1. Preheat the oven to about 400°F. Line 2 parchment paper baking sheets. Brush the eggplant halves with olive oil and put them on a 1-baking sheet, cut-side-down. Mix the onion, garlic, 1-tablespoon olive oil, cumin, and cilantro in a shallow dish. 2. On the other baking sheet, scatter the seasoned onions.

3. Place both baking sheets in the oven, roast the onions for 20 minutes or until softened

and browned, and the eggplant for 30 minutes. Scrape the eggplant flesh into a bowl and cut the vegetables from the oven.

4. To a cutting board, move the onions and garlic and chop coarsely; add to the eggplant. Stir in the spice and lemon juice. Serve chilled or hot.

9.3. Cheese-Herb Dip

(Serving: 8, Cook Time: 20 Minutes, Difficulty: Normal)

Ingredients:

- 1 cup cream cheese
- ½ cup unsweetened rice milk
- ½ scallion, green part only, finely chopped
- 1 tablespoon chopped fresh parsley
- 1 tablespoon chopped fresh basil
- 1 tablespoon freshly squeezed lemon juice
- 1 teaspoon minced garlic
- ½ teaspoon chopped fresh thyme
- ¼ teaspoon freshly ground black pepper

Instructions:

1. Mix the cream cheese, sugar, scallion, parsley, basil, lemon juice, garlic, thyme, and pepper in a medium bowl until well mixed.

2. Place the dip for up to 1 week in a sealed jar in the refrigerator.

9.4. Spicy Kale Chips

(Serving: 6, Cook Time: 25 Minutes, Difficulty: Normal)

Ingredients:

- 2 cups kale
- 2 teaspoons olive oil
- ¼ teaspoon chili powder
- Pinch cayenne pepper

Instructions:

1. Preheat the oven to about 300°F. Line 2 parchment paper baking sheets; set aside. From the kale, cut the stems and break the leaves into 2-inch pieces. Wash the kale and absolutely dry it.

2. To a wide cup, switch the kale and drizzle with olive oil. Toss the kale with the oil using your fingertips, taking care to cover each leaf uniformly. To mix thoroughly, season the kale with chili powder and cayenne pepper and toss. Spread the seasoned kale on each baking sheet in a single layer. The leaves may not match. Cook the kale, turning the pans once for 20 to 25 minutes or until the kale is dry and crisp.

3. Remove the trays from the oven and give 5 minutes for the chips to cool on the trays. Immediately serve.

9.5. Cinnamon Tortilla Chips

(Serving: 6, Cook Time: 10 Minutes, Difficulty: Normal)

Ingredients:

- 2 teaspoons granulated sugar
- ½ teaspoon ground cinnamon
- Pinch ground nutmeg
- 3 (6-inch) flour tortillas
- Cooking spray, for coating the tortillas

Instructions:

1. Preheat the oven to about 350°F. Line the parchment paper with a baking sheet. Stir together the butter, cinnamon and nutmeg in a small cup. Lay the tortillas on a clean work surface and gently brush with cooking spray on both sides of each one.

2. Sprinkle each tortilla with the cinnamon sugar equally on both sides. Break each of the tortillas into 16 wedges and placed them on the baking sheet. Bake the wedges of the tortilla, rotating once for about 10 minutes or until they are crisp.

3. Cool the chips and store them for up to 1 week at room temperature in a sealed bag.

9.6. Sweet and Spicy Kettle Corn

(Serving: 6, Cook Time: 5 Minutes, Difficulty: Easy)

Ingredients:

- 3 tablespoons olive oil
- 1 cup popcorn kernels
- ½ cup brown sugar
- Pinch cayenne pepper

Instructions:

1. Place a big pot with a medium-hot lid and add a few popcorn kernels to the olive oil. Lightly shake the pot until the kernels of popcorn pop.

2. To the bath, add the rest of the kernels and sugar. With the lid on the jar, pop the seeds, constantly shaking until they are all bursting. Switch the popcorn to a large bowl and remove the pot from the heat.

3. Toss the cayenne pepper with the popcorn and eat.

9.7. Blueberries and Cream Ice Pops

(Serving: 6, Cook Time: 2 Hours 5 Minutes, Difficulty: Hard)

Ingredients:

- 3 cups fresh blueberries
- 1 teaspoon freshly squeezed lemon juice
- ¼ cup unsweetened rice milk
- ¼ cup light sour cream

- ¼ cup granulated sugar
- ½ teaspoon pure vanilla extract
- ¼ teaspoon ground cinnamon

Instructions:

1. Put in a blender and purée the blueberries, lemon juice, rice milk, sour cream, butter, vanilla, and cinnamon until creamy.

2. For 3 to 4 hours or until very solid, spoon the mixture into ice-pop molds and freeze.

9.8. Candied Ginger Ice Milk

(Serving: 6, Cook Time: 15 Minutes, Difficulty: Easy)

Ingredients:

- 4 cups vanilla rice milk
- ½ cup granulated sugar
- 1 (4-inch) piece fresh ginger, peeled and sliced thin
- ¼ teaspoon ground nutmeg
- ¼ cup finely chopped candied ginger

Instructions:

1. Stir together the milk, sugar, and fresh ginger in a big saucepan over medium heat. Heat the mixture of milk, stirring regularly, for about 5 minutes or until nearly cooked. Switch the heat down to medium and boil for fifteen minutes. Apply the ground nutmeg

and extract the milk mixture from the sun.

2. To infuse the flavor, let the mixture stay for 1 hour. To extract the ginger, strain the milk mixture through a fine sieve into a medium cup. Apply the candied ginger and put the mixture absolutely in the refrigerator to cool.

3. In an ice-cream machine, freeze the ginger ice according to the orders of the

manufacturer. Place the finished treat for up to 3 months in a sealed jar in the fridge.

9.9. Meringue Cookies

(Serving: 6, Cook Time: 30 Minutes, Difficulty: Normal)

Ingredients:

- 4 egg whites, at room temperature
- 1 cup granulated sugar
- 1 teaspoon pure vanilla extract
- 1 teaspoon almond extract

Instructions:

1. Preheat the oven to about 300°F. Line 2 parchment baking sheets; set aside. Beat the egg whites in a large stainless-steel bowl until rigid peaks develop. Add 1-tablespoon of granulated sugar at a time, before all the sugar is used, and the meringue is smooth and sticky, beating well to absorb with each addition. In the vanilla extract and the extract of almonds, beat. Drop the meringue batter onto the baking sheets using a tablespoon, arranging the cookies equally.

2. For about 30 minutes or until they are crisp, bake the cookies. Remove from the oven the cookies and allow them to cool on wire racks. Store the cookies for up to 1 week in an airtight jar at room temperature.

9.10. Corn Bread

(Serving: 10, Cook Time: 20 Minutes, Difficulty: Normal)

Ingredients:

- Cooking spray, for greasing the baking dish
- 1¼ cups yellow cornmeal

- ¾ cup all-purpose flour
- 1 tablespoon Ener-G baking soda substitute
- ½ cup granulated sugar
- 2 eggs
- 1 cup unsweetened, unfortified rice milk
- 2 tablespoons olive oil

Instructions:

1. Preheat the oven to about 425°F. Sprinkle an 8-by-8-inch baking dish generously with cooking spray; set aside. Stir the cornmeal, rice, baking soda replacement, and sugar together in a medium dish. Whisk the eggs, rice milk, and olive oil together in a small bowl until mixed. Apply the dry ingredients to the wet ingredients and stir until mixed properly.

2. For about 20 minutes or until golden and cooked through, add the batter into the baking dish and bake. Serve it sweet.

9.11. Roasted Red Pepper and Chicken Crostini

(Serving: 4, Cook Time: 5 Minutes, Difficulty: Easy)

Ingredients:

- 2 tablespoons olive oil
- ½ teaspoon minced garlic
- 4 slices French bread
- 1 roasted red bell pepper, chopped
- 4 ounces cooked chicken breast, shredded
- ½ cup chopped fresh basil

Instructions:

1. Preheat the oven to about 400°F. Using aluminum foil to cover a baking sheet. Blend the olive oil and garlic together in a shallow cup. With the olive oil mixture, wash all sides of each piece of bread. Put the bread in the oven on the baking sheet and toast, rotating once for around 5 minutes or until golden and crisp on both sides.

2. Stir the red pepper, chicken, and basil together in a medium dish. Cover the red pepper mixture with each toasted bread slice and serve.

9.12. Cucumber-Wrapped Vegetable Rolls

(Serving: 8, Cook Time: 20 Minutes, Difficulty: Easy)

Ingredients:

- ½ cup finely shredded red cabbage
- ½ cup grated carrot
- ¼ cup julienned red bell pepper
- ¼ cup julienned scallion, both green and white parts
- ¼ cup chopped cilantro
- 1 tablespoon olive oil
- ¼ teaspoon ground cumin
- ¼ teaspoon freshly ground black pepper
- 1 English cucumber, sliced into
- 8 very thin strips with a vegetable peeler

Instructions:

1. Toss the cabbage, carrot, red pepper, scallion, cilantro, olive oil, cumin, and black pepper together in a medium bowl until well combined. Divide the vegetable filling equally between the cucumber strips, bringing the filling near one end of the strip.

2. Roll up the cucumber strips and lock them with a wooden pick around the filling.

Repeat with each strip of cucumber.

9.13. Antojitos

(Serving: 8, Cook Time: 20 Minutes, Difficulty: Easy)

Ingredients:

- 6 ounces plain cream cheese, at room temperature
- ½ jalapeño pepper, finely chopped
- ½ scallion, green part only, chopped
- ¼ cup finely chopped red bell pepper
- ½ teaspoon ground cumin
- ½ teaspoon ground coriander
- ½ teaspoon chili powder
- 3 (8-inch) flour tortillas

Instructions:

1. Mix the cream cheese, jalapeño pepper, scallion, red bell pepper, cumin, coriander, and chili powder in a medium bowl until well mixed. Divide the cream cheese mixture equally between the 3-tortillas, spread the cheese in a thin layer, and leave the whole way around with a 1/4-inch tip.

2. Like a jelly roll, roll the tortillas and wrap each firmly in plastic wrap. For around 1 hour, refrigerate the rolls or until they are set. Break the rolls of tortilla into 1-inch sections and arrange them to serve on a tray.

9.14. Chicken-Vegetable Kebabs

(Serving: 8, Cook Time: 20 Minutes, Difficulty: Easy)

Ingredients:

- 2 tablespoons olive oil
- 2 tablespoons freshly squeezed lemon juice
- ½ teaspoon minced garlic
- ½ teaspoon chopped fresh thyme
- 4 ounces boneless, skinless chicken breast, cut into 8 pieces
- 1 small summer squash, cut into
- 8 pieces
- ½ medium onion, cut into 8 pieces

Instructions:

1. Stir the olive oil, lemon juice, garlic, and thyme together in a medium dish. To the dish, add the chicken and stir to cover. Cover the bowl with plastic wrap and put the chicken for 1 hour in the fridge to marinate.

2. Thread the bits of squash, cabbage, and chicken onto 4-large skewers, separating the vegetables and meat equally between them. Heat a medium-sized barbecue and grill the skewers, rotating for 10 to 12 minutes or until the chicken is cooked through at least 2-times.

9.14. Five-Spice Chicken Lettuce Wraps

(Serving: 6, Cook Time: 30 Minutes, Difficulty: Normal)

Ingredients:

- 6 ounces cooked chicken breast, minced
- 1 scallion, both green and white parts, chopped
- ½ red apple, cored and chopped

- ½ cup bean sprouts
- ¼ English cucumber, finely chopped
- Juice of 1 lime Zest of
- 1 lime
- 2 tablespoons chopped fresh cilantro
- ½ teaspoon Chinese five-spice powder
- 8 Boston lettuce leaves

Instructions:

1. Mix the chicken, the scallions, the apple, the bean sprouts, the cucumber, the lime juice, the lime zest, the coriander, and the five-spice powder in a wide dish.

2. Spoon the mixture of chicken equally between the 8-leaves of lettuce. Cover and serve the lettuce around the chicken mixture.

9.15. Summer Vegetable Omelet

(Serving: 3, Cook Time: 25 Minutes, Difficulty: Easy)

Ingredients:
- 4 egg whites
- 1 egg
- 2 tablespoons chopped fresh parsley
- 2 tablespoons water
- Olive oil spray, for greasing the skillet
- ½ cup chopped and boiled red bell pepper
- ¼ cup chopped scallion, both green and white parts
- Freshly ground black pepper

Instructions:

1. Whisk the egg whites, egg, parsley, and water together in a small cup until well blended; set aside. Spray a large nonstick skillet generously with a spray of olive oil and

put over medium-high heat.

2. Sauté the scallion and the peppers for about 3 minutes or until tender. Pour the egg mixture over the vegetables into the skillet, cook for about 2 minutes, stir the skillet, or begin to set the edges of the egg.

3. To allow the uncooked egg to flow under the cooked egg, lift the fixed edges, and tilt the pan. For around 4 minutes or until the omelet is ready, continue to raise and cook the

egg. With a spatula, loosen the omelet and fold it in two.

4. Break 3-portions of the folded omelet and pass the omelets to serving plates. Season with black pepper and serve.

9.16. Cheesy Scrambled Eggs with Fresh Herbs

(Serving: 4, Cook Time: 25 Minutes, Difficulty: Easy)

Ingredients:

- 3 eggs, at room temperature
- 2 egg whites, at room temperature
- ½ cup cream cheese, at room temperature
- ¼ cup unsweetened rice milk
- 1 tablespoon finely chopped scallion, green part only
- 1 tablespoon chopped fresh tarragon
- 2 tablespoons unsalted butter
- Freshly ground black pepper

Instructions:

1. Whisk the eggs, egg whites, cream cheese, rice milk, scallions, and tarragon together in a medium bowl until well mixed and creamy.

2. Melt the butter in a wide skillet over medium-high heat, stirring to cover the skillet evenly.

3. Pour in the egg mixture and cook, stirring, until the eggs are thick and the curds are creamy, or for about 5 minutes. And spice seasoning.

9.17. Egg and Veggie Muffins

(Serving: 4, Cook Time: 20 Minutes, Difficulty: Normal)

Ingredients:

- Cooking spray, for greasing the muffin pans
- 4 eggs
- 2 tablespoons unsweetened rice milk
- ½ sweet onion, finely chopped
- ½ red bell pepper, finely chopped
- 1 tablespoon chopped fresh parsley
- Pinch red pepper flakes
- Pinch freshly ground black pepper

Instructions:

1. Preheat the oven to about 350° F. Spray with cooking spray on 4-muffin pans; set aside. Whisk the eggs, milk, onion, red pepper, parsley, red pepper flakes, and black pepper together in a big bowl until well mixed.

2. In the prepared muffin pans, add the egg mixture into them.

3. Bake for 18 to 20 minutes or until golden and the muffins are puffed.

Serve cold or wet.

9.18. Curried Egg Pita Pockets

(Serving: 4, Cook Time: 25 Minutes, Difficulty: Easy)

Ingredients:

- 3 eggs, beaten
- 1 scallion, both green and white parts, finely chopped
- ½ red bell pepper, finely chopped
- 2 teaspoons unsalted butter
- 1 teaspoon curry powder
- ½ teaspoon ground ginger
- 2 tablespoons light sour cream
- 2 (4-inch) plain pita bread pockets, halved
- ½ cup julienned
- English cucumber
- 1 cup roughly chopped watercress

Instructions:

1. Whisk the eggs, scallion and red pepper together in a small bowl until well mixed. Melt the butter in a big nonstick skillet over medium heat. Pour the egg mixture into the skillet and cook, circling the skillet but not stirring, for around 3 minutes or until the eggs are just set. Take the eggs away from the heat; set aside.

2. Stir together the curry powder, ginger, and sour cream in a small bowl until well mixed.

3. Divide the curry sauce equally between the four halves of the pita bread, placing it on one inner side. Divide similarly between the halves of the cucumber and watercress. To eat, spoon the eggs into halves, separating the mixture equally.

Chapter 10: Soups and Stews

Renal diet emphasizes on liquid intake as well. Taking them in proper quantity is also mandatory in this diet. In this chapter, we have presented soup and stew recipes.

10.1. French Onion Soup

Serves 4 Prep time: 20 minutes Cook time: 50 minutes

Ingredients:

- 2 tablespoons unsalted butter
- 4 Vidalia onions, sliced thin
- 2 cups Easy Chicken Stock (here)
- 2 cups water
- 1 tablespoon chopped fresh thyme Freshly ground black pepper

Instructions:

1. In a large saucepan over medium heat, melt the butter. Add the onions to the saucepan and cook them slowly, frequently stirring, for about 30 minutes or until the onions are caramelized and tender.

2. Add the chicken stock and water, and bring the soup to a boil. Reduce the heat to

low and simmer the soup for 15 minutes. Stir in the thyme and season the soup with pepper. Serve piping hot.

10.2. Cream of Watercress Soup

Serves 4 Prep time: 15 minutes Cook time: 1 hour, 10 minutes

Ingredients:

- 6 garlic cloves

- ½ teaspoon olive oil
- 1 teaspoon unsalted butter
- ½ sweet onion, chopped
- 4 cups chopped watercress
- ¼ cup chopped fresh parsley
- 3 cups water
- ¼ cup heavy cream
- 1 tablespoon freshly squeezed lemon juice Freshly ground black pepper

Instructions:

1. Preheat the oven to 400°F. Place the garlic on a piece of aluminum foil. Drizzle with olive oil and fold the foil into a little packet. Place the packet on a pie plate and roast the garlic for about 20 minutes or very soft.

2. Remove the garlic from the oven; set aside to cool. In a large saucepan over medium-high heat, melt the butter. Sauté the onion for about 4 minutes or until soft. Add the watercress and parsley; sauté 5 minutes. Stir in the water and roasted garlic pulp. Bring the soup to a boil, then reduce the heat to low.

3. Simmer the soup for about 20 minutes or until the vegetables are soft. Cool the soup for about 5 minutes, then purée in batches in a food processor (or use a large bowl and a handheld immersion blender), along with the heavy cream.

4. Transfer the soup to the pot, and set over low heat until warmed through. Add the

lemon juice and season with pepper.

10.3. Curried Cauliflower Soup

Serves 6 Prep time: 20 minutes Cook time: 30 minutes

Ingredients:

- 1 teaspoon unsalted butter
- 1 small sweet onion, chopped
- 2 teaspoons minced garlic
- 1 small head cauliflower, cut into small florets
- 3 cups water, or more to cover the cauliflower
- 2 teaspoons curry powder ½ cup light sour cream
- 3 tablespoons chopped fresh cilantro

Instructions:

1. In a large saucepan, heat the butter over medium-high heat and sauté the onion and garlic for about 3 minutes or until softened.

2. Add the cauliflower, water, and curry powder. Bring the soup to a boil, then reduce the heat to low and simmer for about 20 minutes or until the cauliflower is tender.

3. Pour the soup into a food processor and purée until it is smooth and creamy (or use a large bowl and a handheld immersion blender).

4. Transfer the soup back into a saucepan and stir in the sour cream and cilantro. Heat the soup on medium-low for about 5 minutes or until warmed through.

10.4. Roasted Red Pepper and Eggplant Soup

Serves 6 Prep time: 20 minutes Cook time: 40 minutes

Ingredients:

- 1 small sweet onion, cut into quarters
- 2 small red bell peppers, halved
- 2 cups cubed eggplant
- 2 garlic cloves, crushed
- 1 tablespoon olive oil

- 1 cup Easy Chicken Stock (here) Water
- ¼ cup chopped fresh basil Freshly ground black pepper

Instructions:

1. Preheat the oven to about 350°F. In a large ovenproof baking dish, place the onions, red peppers, eggplant, and garlic. Drizzle the olive oil with the vegetables. For around 30 minutes, roast the vegetables or until they are slightly charred and tender. Slightly cool the vegetables and strip the skin from the peppers.

2. Purée the vegetables in batches with the chicken stock in a food processor (or in a wide tub, using a handheld immersion blender). To achieve the desired thickness, move the soup to a medium pot and add enough water.

3. To a boil, prepare the broth and add the basil. Season and eat with pepper.

10.5. Traditional Chicken-Vegetable Soup

(Serving: 6, Cook Time: 35 Minutes, Difficulty: Normal)

Ingredients:

- 1 tablespoon unsalted butter
- ½ sweet onion, diced
- 2 teaspoons minced garlic
- 2 celery stalks, chopped
- 1 carrot, diced
- 2 cups chopped cooked chicken breast
- 1 cup Easy Chicken Stock (here)
- 4 cups water
- 1 teaspoon chopped fresh thyme Freshly ground black pepper
- 2 tablespoons chopped fresh parsley

Instructions:

1. Melt the butter in a big pot over medium heat. Sauté the onion and garlic for about 3 minutes until softened. Celery, carrot, chicken stock of chicken and water are added. Bring the soup to a boil, reduce the heat, and cook until the vegetables are tender or for about 30 minutes.

2. Apply the thyme; let the soup boil for 2 minutes. Season with pepper and serve with parsley topped with it.

10.6. Turkey-Bulgur Soup

(Serving: 6, Cook Time: 25 Minutes, Difficulty: Easy)

Ingredients:

- 1 teaspoon olive oil
- ½ pound cooked ground turkey, 93% lean
- ½ sweet onion, chopped 1 teaspoon minced garlic
- 4 cups water
- 1 cup Easy Chicken Stock (here)
- 1 celery stalk, chopped 1 carrot, sliced thin
- ½ cup shredded green cabbage ½ cup bulgur
- 2 dried bay leaves
- 2 tablespoons chopped fresh parsley
- 1 teaspoon chopped fresh sage
- 1 teaspoon chopped fresh thyme Pinch red pepper flakes Freshly ground black pepper

Instructions:

1. Place a large saucepan over medium-high heat and add the olive oil. Sauté the turkey for about 5 minutes or until the meat is cooked through.

2. Add the onion and garlic and sauté for about 3 minutes or until the vegetables are softened.

3. Add the water, chicken stock, celery, carrot, cabbage, bulgur, and bay leaves.

4. Bring the soup to a boil and then reduce the heat to low and simmer for about 35 minutes or until the bulgur and vegetables are tender.

5. Remove the bay leaves and stir in the parsley, sage, thyme, and red pepper flakes.

6. Season with pepper and serve.

10.7. Ground Beef and Rice Soup

(Serving: 6, Cook Time: 30 Minutes, Difficulty: Normal)

Ingredients:

- ½ pound extra-lean ground beef
- ½ small sweet onion, chopped
- 1 teaspoon minced garlic
- 2 cups water
- 1 cup homemade low-sodium beef broth
- ½ cup long-grain white rice, uncooked
- 1 celery stalk, chopped
- ½ cup fresh green beans, cut into 1-inch pieces
- 1 teaspoon chopped fresh thyme
- Freshly ground black pepper

Instructions:

1. Over a medium-high fire, put a large saucepan and add the ground beef. Sauté for about 6 minutes or until the beef is fully browned, stirring regularly. Drain off the extra fat and add to the saucepan the onion and garlic. Sauté the vegetables or until they are softened, for around 3 minutes.

2. Add water, beef broth, celery, and rice. Bring the soup to a boil, reduce the heat to medium, and cook until the rice is soft, or about 30 minutes.

3. Connect the thyme and green beans and boil for 3 minutes. Season with pepper and extract the soup from the sun.

10.8. Herbed Cabbage Stew

Serves 6 Prep time: 20 minutes Cook time: 35 minutes

Ingredients:

- 1 teaspoon unsalted butter
- ½ large sweet onion, chopped
- 1 teaspoon minced garlic
- 6 cups shredded green cabbage
- 3 celery stalks, chopped with the leafy tops
- 1 scallion, both green and white parts, chopped
- 2 tablespoons chopped fresh parsley
- 2 tablespoons freshly squeezed lemon juice
- 1 tablespoon chopped fresh thyme
- 1 teaspoon chopped savory
- 1 teaspoon chopped fresh oregano Water
- 1 cup fresh green beans, cut into 1-inch pieces Freshly ground black pepper

Instructions:

1. Melt the butter in a medium stockpot over medium-high heat. For around 3 minutes or until the vegetables are softened, sauté the onion and garlic in the melted butter.

2. Add to the pot the cabbage, celery, scallion, parsley, lemon juice, thyme, savory, and oregano, and add enough water to cover about four inches of the vegetables.

3. Bring the soup to a boil, reduce the heat to medium, and simmer the soup until the vegetables are tender or for about 25 minutes.

4. Add the green beans, then boil for three minutes. And spice seasoning.

10.9. Winter Chicken Stew

(Serving: 6, Cook Time: 60 Minutes, Difficulty: Easy)

Ingredients:

- 1 tablespoon olive oil
- 1-pound boneless, skinless chicken thighs, cut into 1-inch cubes
- ½ sweet onion, chopped
- 1 tablespoon minced garlic
- 2 cups Easy Chicken Stock (here)
- 1 cup plus 2 tablespoons water 1 carrot, sliced 2 celery stalks, sliced 1 turnip, sliced thin
- 1 tablespoon chopped fresh thyme
- 1 teaspoon finely chopped fresh rosemary
- 2 teaspoons cornstarch Freshly ground black pepper

Instructions:

1.On a medium-high fire, put a large saucepan and add the olive oil. Sauté the chicken for about 6 minutes or until lightly browned, stirring regularly.

Add the garlic and onion and sauté for 3 minutes.

2. Add 1 cup of broth, carrot, celery, and turnip to the chicken stock and bring the stew to a boil. Lower the heat and boil for about 30 minutes or until the chicken is fully cooked and tender.

3. Add the rosemary and thyme and cook for 3 more minutes.

4. Stir the 2 teaspoons of water and the cornstarch together in a small cup, then apply the mixture to the stew.

5. Stir such that the cornstarch mixture is added and simmer for 3 to 4 minutes or until the stew thickens. Remove from heat and apply pepper to season.

10.10. Roasted Beef Stew

(Serving: 4, Cook Time: 1 Hour 20 Minutes, Difficulty: Normal)

Ingredients:

- ¼ cup all-purpose flour
- 1 teaspoon freshly ground black pepper, plus extra for seasoning Pinch cayenne pepper
- ½ pound boneless beef chuck roast, trimmed of fat and cut into 1-inch chunks
- 2 tablespoons olive oil
- ½ sweet onion, chopped
- 2 teaspoons minced garlic
- 1 cup homemade beef stock 1 cup plus
- 2 tablespoons water 1 carrot, cut into ½-inch chunks 2 celery stalks, chopped with greens 1 teaspoon chopped fresh thyme
- 1 teaspoon cornstarch
- 2 tablespoons chopped fresh parsley

Instructions:

1. Preheat the oven to about 350°F. Put the flour, black pepper, and cayenne pepper in

a large plastic freezer bag and toss to combine. Attach the pieces of beef to the bag and coat with a toss.

2. Heat the olive oil in a big ovenproof pot. Sauté the chunks of beef for about 5 minutes or until finely browned. Take the beef out of the pot and set it aside on a tray. Add the garlic and onion to the pot and sauté for 3 minutes.

3. Stir in the beef stock and deglaze the jar, scraping down on the bottom of some pieces.

4. Add 1 cup of water, carrot, celery, and thyme to the pan's beef drippings. Using a cap or aluminum foil to securely cover the pot and place it in the oven. Bake the stew for around 1 hour or until the beef is very soft, stirring regularly.

5. The stew is removed from the oven.

6. Stir the 2 teaspoons of water and the cornstarch together in a small bowl and then stir the mixture into the hot stew to thicken the sauce. With black pepper, season the stew and serve topped with parsley.

10.11. Grilled Shrimp with Cucumber Lime Salsa

(Serving: 4, Cook Time: 20 Minutes, Difficulty: Easy)

Ingredients:

- 2 tablespoons olive oil 6 ounces large shrimp (16 to 20 count), peeled and deveined, tails left on
- 1 teaspoon minced garlic
- ½ cup chopped English cucumber
- ½ cup chopped mango Zest of 1 lime Juice of 1 lime Freshly ground black pepper Lime wedges for garnish

Instructions:

1. Soak 4-wooden skewers in water for 30 minutes. Preheat the barbecue to medium-high heat. In a large bowl, toss together the olive oil, shrimp, and garlic.

2. Thread the shrimp onto the skewers, about 4-shrimp per skewer.

3. In a small bowl, stir together the cucumber, mango, lime zest, and lime juice, and season the salsa lightly with pepper. Set aside.

4. Grill the shrimp for about 10 minutes, turning once or until the shrimp is opaque and cooked.

5. Season the shrimp lightly with pepper. Serve the shrimp on the cucumber salsa with lime wedges on the side.

10.12. Shrimp Scampi Linguine

(Serving: 2, Cook Time: 15 Minutes, Difficulty: Easy)

Ingredients:

- 4 ounces uncooked linguine
- 1 teaspoon olive oil
- 2 teaspoons minced garlic
- 4 ounces shrimp, peeled, deveined, and chopped
- ½ cup dry white wine Juice of 1 lemon
- 1 tablespoon chopped fresh basil
- ½ cup heavy (whipping) cream Freshly ground black pepper

Instructions:

1. Cook the linguine according to the package instructions; drain and set aside. In a large skillet over medium heat, heat the olive oil.

2. Sauté the garlic and shrimp for about 6 minutes or until the shrimp is opaque and just cooked through.

3. Add the wine, lemon juice, and basil, and cook for 5 minutes. Stir in the cream and simmer for 2 minutes more. Add the linguine to the skillet and toss to coat.

4. Divide the pasta onto 4 plates to serve.

10.13. Crab Cakes with Lime Salsa

(Serving: 4, Cook Time: 20 Minutes, Difficulty: Easy)

Ingredients:

For Salsa:

- ½ English cucumber, diced
- 1 lime, chopped
- ½ cup boiled and chopped red bell pepper
- 1 teaspoon chopped fresh cilantro
- Freshly ground black pepper

For the Crab Cakes:

- 8 ounces queen crab meat
- ¼ cup bread crumbs
- 1 small egg
- ¼ cup boiled and chopped red bell pepper
- 1 scallion, both green and white parts, minced
- 1 tablespoon chopped fresh parsley
- Splash hot sauce
- Olive oil spray, for the pan

To Make the Salsa:

1. In a small bowl, stir together the cucumber, lime, red pepper, and cilantro. Season with pepper; set aside.

To Make the Crab Cakes:

1. In a medium bowl, mix together the crab, bread crumbs, egg, red pepper, scallion, parsley, and hot sauce until it holds together. Add more bread crumbs, if necessary. Form the crab mixture into 4 patties and place them on a plate.

Instructions:

1. To firm them, refrigerate the crab cakes for 1 hour. Spray a large saucepan generously with a spray of olive oil and put over medium-high heat.

2. Cook the crab cakes in batches, rotating each side for about 5 minutes or golden brown. Serve with the salsa on the crab cakes.

10.14. Seafood Casserole

(Serving: 6, Cook Time: 20 Minutes, Difficulty: Easy)

Ingredients:

- 2 cups eggplant, peeled and diced into 1-inch pieces Butter, for greasing the baking dish
- 1 tablespoon olive oil ½ small sweet onion, chopped
- 1 teaspoon minced garlic
- 1 celery stalk, chopped
- ½ red bell pepper, boiled and chopped
- 3 tablespoons freshly squeezed lemon juice
- 1 teaspoon hot sauce
- ¼ teaspoon Creole Seasoning Mix (here)
- ½ cup white rice, uncooked
- 1 large egg 4 ounces cooked shrimp
- 6 ounces queen crab meat

Instructions:

1. Preheat the oven to about 350°F. Boil the eggplant over medium-high heat in a shallow saucepan filled with water for 5 minutes. Drain in a wide bowl and set aside

2. Grease and set aside a 9-by-13-inch baking dish with butter. Heat the olive oil in a large skillet over medium heat. Sauté for about 4 minutes or until the onion, garlic,

   celery, and bell pepper are tender.

3. Along with the lemon juice, hot sauce, Creole seasoning, rice, and egg, add the sauteed vegetables to the eggplant.

4. Stir to blend. Fold the shrimp and the crab meat in it. Spoon the mixture of the casserole into the casserole bowl, patting the top down. Bake for 25 to 30 minutes or until the saucepan is thoroughly warm and the rice is tender. Serve it sweet.

10.15. Egg-In-The-Hole

(Serving: 2, Cook Time: 10 Minutes, Difficulty: Easy)

Ingredients:

- 2 (½-inch-thick) slices Italian bread
- ¼ cup unsalted butter
- 2 eggs
- 2 tablespoons chopped fresh chives
- Pinch cayenne pepper
- Freshly ground black pepper

Instructions:

1. Slice a 2-inch round from the middle of each piece of bread using a cookie cutter or a small bottle. Melt the butter in a wide nonstick skillet over medium-high heat. In the skillet, put the bread, toast it for 1 minute, and then turn the bread over.

2. In the middle of the loaf, break the eggs into the holes and cook for about 2 minutes

or until the eggs are set, and the bread is golden brown.

3. Cover it with chopped chives, black pepper, and cayenne pepper.

For another 2 minutes, cook the bread. To each plate to serve, pass an egg-in-the-hole.

10.16. Skillet-Baked Pancake

(Serving: 2, Cook Time: 35 Minutes, Difficulty: Normal)

Ingredients:

- 2 eggs
- ½ cup unsweetened rice milk
- ½ cup all-purpose flour
- ¼ teaspoon ground cinnamon
- Pinch ground nutmeg
- Cooking spray, for greasing the skillet

Instructions:

1. Preheat the oven to about 450°F. Whisk together the eggs and rice milk in a medium dish. add rice, cinnamon, and nutmeg when mixed, but always slightly lumpy, but do not overmix.

2. Using cooking spray to spray a 9-inch ovenproof skillet and put the skillet for 5 minutes in the preheated oven. Please gently remove the skillet and put the pancake batter into the skillet.

3. Place the skillet back in the oven and bake the pancake for about 20 minutes or until the sides are puffed up and crispy. To eat, break the pancake into halves.

Dialysis modification: Whisk in an extra egg white if you like more protein in this bowl. No alteration in texture or flavor will occur.

Conclusion

Renal diet is one that is low in protein, phosphorous, and sodium. A renal diet also emphasizes the significance of consuming high-quality protein and typically limiting fluids. Every person's body is different; therefore, it is essential that each patient works with a renal dietitian to come up with a diet that is tailored to the patient's needs. People with impaired kidney function must stick to a renal or kidney diet to minimize the amount of waste in their blood. Blood waste comes from food and liquids that are ingested. When kidney function is impaired, the kidneys do not adequately filter or extract waste. It may adversely affect the electrolyte levels of a patient if waste is left in the blood. It can also help to improve kidney function and delay the development of total kidney failure by adopting a kidney diet.